Nutritional Pilates

Relieve Joint Pain, Lose Unwanted Weight, and Prevent Chronic Disease to Become Your Most Vibrant Self!

Katrina Foe

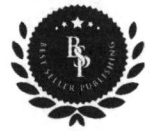

Copyright © 2023 by Katrina Foe

All rights reserved. No part of this book may be used or reproduced in any manner whatsoever without prior written consent of the author, except as provided by the United States of America copyright law.

Published by Best Seller Publishing®, St. Augustine, FL
Best Seller Publishing® is a registered trademark.
Printed in the United States of America.

ISBN: _____

This publication is designed to provide accurate and authoritative information with regard to the subject matter covered. It is sold with the understanding that the publisher is not engaged in rendering legal, accounting, or other professional advice. If legal advice or other expert assistance is required, the services of a competent professional should be sought. The opinions expressed by the author in this book are not endorsed by Best Seller Publishing® and are the sole responsibility of the author rendering the opinion.

For more information, please write:
Best Seller Publishing®
53 Marine Street
St. Augustine, FL 32084
or call 1 (626) 765-9750
Visit us online at: www.BestSellerPublishing.org

Praise for the Author

"Katrina Foe is a uniquely talented, skillful and dedicated health educator focused on the intersection of movement and functional nutrition. This powerful combination enhances vitality, clarity and confidence."

—Elizabeth Larkam, author of
Fascia in Motion, Handspring Publishing

"With her decades of experience, Katrina brilliantly weaves together the potency of these two modalities to provide a valuable resource at your fingertips. If you're interested in optimizing your health, this book is a must have."

—Tiffany Cruikshank, LAc, MAOM, author of
Optimal Health for a Vibrant Life and
founder of Yoga Medicine®

"Katrina Foe NCPT, BCHN, MRWP is a wealth of knowledge and experience in the field of nutrition and Pilates. She knows the importance of incorporating these things into her clients' lifestyles to help maintain health and helping to aid in preventing disease. She believes in the keto and low carb lifestyle as an option to help her clients improve their overall health. In my opinion, we need many more practitioners out there like her who understand the importance of incorporating all of these things as a way to improve overall health, especially as the rates of cancer, diabetes and other diseases are on the rise."

—Christine Moore, FNTP,
Certified Totalfit Level 1 Coach, author of
*Real Food Keto: Applying Nutritional
Therapy to Your Low-Carb, High-Fat Diet*

Dedication

This book is dedicated to my seven precious children. People ask me all the time how in the world I get everything done that I do with seven children. And I ask, how in the world do you get anything done without seven children?

You guys redefine what love and support look like for me. I pray that the principles in this book will be deeply embedded into your hearts, so that we can break the generational curse of chronic disease in our family.

Contents

FOREWORD BY NORA ST. JOHN, MS 1
FOREWORD BY MARGARET FLOYD BARRY, FNTP, MRWP, CGP 3
PROLOGUE 7
INTRODUCTION 9
    Recipe for Chronic Disease 13
1 YOUR POSTURE HANGS IN THE (MUSCLE) BALANCE 17
    So, What Is Pilates? 18
    Coming Back to the "Why" 19
    Pilates' Little Secret 21
    Perfecting Your Posture 25
2 WHEN YOU'RE THROWN OFF BALANCE, FIND YOUR
    IMBALANCES 33
    The Top Five Muscle Imbalances 34
    Spotting Additional Balance Issues 51
    Is There Such a Thing as "Good" Pain? 51
    Three Steps to Balancing Muscle Imbalances 53
    A Little About Cardiovascular Exercise 55
3 THE SURPRISING EFFECTS OF INSULIN 59
    Everything We've Been Taught About Dieting Is Wrong ... 60

	What Insulin Does to Our Bodies	61
	Managing Insulin Spikes	63
	Processed Carbohydrates in the Modern Diet	68
4	**HEADING OFF CHRONIC DISEASE AT THE PASS**	**73**
	Extra Weight and a Bigger Problem	73
	The Chronic Disease Spectrum	74
	Chronic Diseases to Avoid	77
5	**THE IMPORTANCE OF DIET**	**87**
	Our Ongoing Love Affair with Carbs	88
	Putting a Low Carb Plan into Action	90
	Good Fats vs. Bad Fats	91
	Measuring Your Intake	96
	Jamie's Carb Epiphany	100
6	**PROBLEM-SOLVING WITH A LOW INSULIN DIET**	**103**
	The Dilemma of Fat Digestion	103
	Electrolytes and the Keto Flu	106
	The Skinny on Sweeteners	107
	Bio-Individuality and Food Sensitivity	110
	It's All About Timing	111
	The Importance of Food Quality	112
7	**THE IMPACT OF GENETICS**	**117**
	How Much Do Your Genes Affect Your Health?	118
8	**GO WITH YOUR GUT**	**123**
	How the Digestive System Works	124
	Doing the Healing Work	132
	The End of the Digestive Journey	133
	A Client's Digestion Is Back on Track	136
9	**HORMONES**	**139**
	How the Thyroid Works	140
	Cortisol, Sleep, and Stress	144
	The Process for Regulating Sex Hormones	147

10 TALKING ABOUT TOXINS	153
Becoming Toxin Detectives	153
Other Forms of Toxins	155
11 QUESTIONS TO GUIDE YOU ON YOUR JOURNEY	161
Five Questions to Get You on Your Way	162
CONCLUSION	171
ABOUT THE AUTHOR	177

Foreword
by Nora St. John, MS

> Physical fitness is the first requisite of happiness.
> —Joseph H. Pilates

Joseph Pilates brought "Contrology," his method of physical and mental conditioning, to America in the 1920s. His emphasis on the mind-body connection was decades ahead of most other physical fitness techniques, and his influence and ideas have continued to grow over the last century. Pilates is a low-impact but highly effective movement technique known to decrease low back pain, improve balance, and increase functional capacity for clients at any stage of life. It is used for rehabilitation, general conditioning, and enhancing athletic performance and has grown into a worldwide fitness phenomenon, with instructors and practitioners in over 150 countries.

Joseph Pilates brought into focus the importance of the connection between mind and body. Katrina Foe, a Pilates instructor and educator with over twenty years' experience, is taking the mind-body connection one step further by adding nutritional insights to our understanding of true physical fitness. If Joseph Pilates emphasized how we move and how we think, Katrina is adding what we eat as a third pillar of physical fitness. Her strong background in science, anatomy, nutrition, and health have led her to explore nutrition in-depth and to incorporate it with Pilates into a robust, whole body training program that can transform your life from the inside out.

Katrina does not come to this work with a purely theoretical approach. She has truly walked the talk. In the world of movement, Katrina has run a very successful studio, taught clients of all kinds, trained Pilates instructors for almost twenty years, and developed educational workshops, programs, and resources that are exceptionally effective. Along the way Katrina has been raising her seven children and using nutrition to maintain and optimize the health and well-being of her family. She has personally used food as a tool for managing both mental and physical health and for combating and overcoming serious health issues.

I have known Katrina as an educator and Pilates practitioner for over fifteen years, and I am delighted to support her integration of mind-body wellness with the powerful tool of nutrition for lifelong health and vitality.

Be well and take care,

—Nora St. John, MS
Education Program Director
Balanced Body Education

Foreword
by Margaret Floyd Barry, FNTP, MRWP, CGP

I first met Katrina Foe as a student in our advanced practitioner training program, Restorative Wellness Solutions. She was hungry for better information and more tools and had a passion for learning and health that was contagious.

In my role as Owner and Executive Director of this program, I've seen a lot of practitioners come and go, and I've noted that there are several different types of health professional. There are those who struggle with new concepts, tend to get overwhelmed quickly, and just squeeze by in the end. There are those who dig in and get a solid working understanding of the concepts with a lot of hard work. And then there are those who just seem to "get it"; they're implementing new tools and ideas as soon as they learn them and can't wait to share with others. Katrina is one of these latter types: a natural.

Perhaps what makes Katrina such a natural is her own extensive personal experience with extreme health challenges. Diagnosed with breast cancer after the birth of her fifth child, she refused to accept this as her fate and bravely chose the path less trodden. She turned away from the invasive and damaging treatments the medical world had to offer, and instead dove into the research to understand the disease process at play in her body, the combination of internal and external factors that allowed the cancer to grow, and how best to reverse this situation in a way that worked in concert with her body, not against it.

And that's exactly what she did. Katrina put her breast cancer into remission entirely through holistic strategies: manipulating her diet, healing her gut, detoxifying her body, and ensuring that her physiology was set up to thrive. She has now transformed this challenging personal experience into an opportunity to help others in their journey. Many of the tools and concepts she's going to teach you here in this book are the very ones she used in her own healing process.

In 2020, Katrina joined our teaching team at Restorative Wellness Solutions and now trains and mentors other practitioners in these same tools that were so profound for her healing and in her clinical practice. As a homeschooling mom of seven, running a Pilates studio, a thriving Pilates teacher training program, and a thriving nutrition practice, you'd think she has her plate full—but this is Katrina: wanting to pay it forward and share what she's learned with other practitioners so that these tools can be used far and wide.

What inspires and impresses me most about Katrina, however, isn't even this incredible commitment to living what she teaches and overcoming daunting health challenges. It's the warrior inside her that refuses to settle. She's not afraid to fight for what she believes in and to ask the hard questions when something doesn't make sense. She doesn't take things at face value and isn't afraid to challenge when something doesn't sit right. She's not attached to one position or perspective—she's always open to learning something new and incorporating that into how she lives, works, and guides others.

These qualities are exactly what you want in someone who will guide you to your own personal potential.

What I know about Katrina is that she is relentless in her pursuit of knowledge about the healing process and equally dogged in sharing what she's learned, whether that be through her private nutrition practice, in her Pilates studio, or while training other health professionals with the very tools that have been so integral to her own healing. She's not afraid to fight for her clients' health and holds a vision of what's possible for you and your health that is likely beyond what you've even considered within reach.

With this book in your hands, you get to enjoy the fruits of Katrina's journey and follow her road map to truly optimizing your health. Dig in, follow her advice, and watch your physical well-being rise to a whole new level as a result.

—Margaret Floyd Barry, FNTP, MRWP, CGP
Owner and Executive Director, Restorative Wellness Solutions (www.restorativewellnesssolutions.com)
Owner, The Eat Naked Kitchen
(www.eatnakedkitchen.com)
Author of *Eat Naked: Unprocessed, Unpolluted and Undressed Eating for a Healthier, Sexier You* and *The Naked Foods Cookbook*

Prologue

Guiding clients through this work, I have identified three types of people. And I want you to see which one you identify with the most.

The first individual is the frugal DIY person who reads books like this and does the entire thing on their own. They may need to do some additional research and digging, but they're very scrappy and they're going to figure things out all by themselves. They don't need someone else to help them or answer questions, and frankly, they don't really want someone else to get in the way.

The second individual needs help because they know that they won't stay the course on their own. They have lots of questions, and they want someone to be there to answer them. They want someone to have scheduled meetings with to discuss the plan, or maybe even create one for them.

The third person (like myself) wants to become a practitioner and pay it forward. They want to understand the entirety of what is going on and pull the curtain back. They want not only to heal themselves but also to spread the message to help others heal. This person is inspired by learning and growing;

they are not content with just getting it done and moving on. They want to empower others and see the looks on their clients' faces when their clients learn that they too can heal. Yes, they may get a whole new career out of it, but they do this because they are passionate about spreading the word.

All three types of people can be successful in changing the trajectory of their health—they're just doing it in different ways.

Which one are you?

Introduction

There's more.

That's the message of this book. There are more options than the current standard of care offerings to feel better and find your vibrance.

Our medical model seeks to mask any uncomfortable symptoms, but that shouldn't be the goal. We need to optimize our bodies and make sure everything is functioning at the best level it can, but currently, the bar is too low.

In 2015, I was nursing my fifth child when I found a large, golf ball-sized lump. At that time I had mastitis, so I was not very concerned because I thought that it was just part of the nursing process.

However, when the mastitis resolved and the lump was still there, my curiosity was piqued. It turned out it was the dreaded "C" word.

I had to decide how I would handle it, but I had questions. How in the world did this happen to me? At the time, I was thirty-eight, and I felt fine. Our family had been working on our health fairly aggressively and had made great progress. Heck, we had even moved out to the country to raise our own grass-finished meat. We had gotten processed food out of our lives and were doing intensive work on our guts. It seemed inconceivable that this would happen to someone like me.

I was scared, and I felt very alone. I had always thought that I would get heart disease because three out of four of my grandparents had died of it, but what I didn't know was that my grandmother had had breast cancer, and my dad, prostate cancer twice. This was not discussed in my family, bizarrely enough.

I wondered if there was anything wrong with my diet and lifestyle. I decided to clean the slate of everything I thought I knew and dive into discovering what was helpful for cancer prevention and remission. I needed to reexamine everything that I was doing and eating because clearly something wasn't working. It is a very confusing world out there when you're trying to do your research because you can find someone to say whatever you want to hear, and it's almost impossible to know who to trust.

I started my journey by going to Mexico to a Gerson cancer clinic. I had read the clinic's books but did not fully understand the *why* behind what they recommended, like removing salt from my diet, removing all fat (except for a tablespoon of flaxseed oil per day), and taking thyroid medication when they hadn't even tested my thyroid numbers.

By the third day, the director of the facility sat me down and said, "You need to just trust in the process." But I still had questions that weren't answered.

I replied, "This is my life we're talking about, not just a beauty treatment."

He responded by telling me that if I couldn't just trust in the process, I needed to leave.

Yes, I got kicked out of a cancer clinic.

This rocked my world. I'm inquisitive by nature—I want to fully understand all the nuances of something. As a teacher, I know to always welcome questions because I know that the people who are really engaging in the material will naturally have questions come up as they dig into it and apply it to real life. I was fascinated by the process in such an intense way because my life was at stake, and I was going to do everything I could to get to the bottom of why this had happened to me. I didn't buy the standard answer that doctors usually give—that it "just happens." I called BS on that.

Everyone in the cancer world at that time was talking about raw vegan diets, so my husband and I did a twenty-one-day juice fast. By the time it was over, we felt like we were going to eat each other, which I now know was because it had seriously messed up our blood sugar.

Yes, I eventually healed my breast cancer naturally—I had no surgery, radiation, or chemo. But what I discovered along my journey was shocking and frustrating.

I learned that there are many symptoms that point toward dysfunction and will eventually lead to chronic disease. If you don't address them, you're going to end up with big, bad scary illnesses, like heart disease, diabetes, cancer, or dementia. If you do address them, not only will you avoid those huge potholes, but you're also going to feel better as a side benefit.

I firmly believe that there is no such thing as a hypochondriac; when someone is labeled this way, it's really just a matter of a practitioner who doesn't have the answers. I'm fine not having all the answers—it challenges me to dig in deeper.

Too many practitioners are complacent. Their training is outdated, and they don't have the time to keep up on the current research. They don't have the clinical experience to know that chronic disease is preventable and even reversible.

I don't blame this on the practitioners, who are generally well meaning, as much as the insurance companies that dictate how much time they get with a client and what they will cover. However, putting cancer in remission is hard work that there isn't a magic pill for. To prevent and reverse disease, you're going against the grain—not only of what your body is used to, but also against what society says is acceptable.

> Putting cancer in remission is hard work that there isn't a magic pill for.

The insurance industry doesn't allow practitioners the time to do this hard work with their clients—they barely get fifteen minutes per person, so it's much easier to give the client a pill and send them on their way. But this doesn't fix the problem; it's simply a Band-Aid that is going to allow the real issue to continue to fester until it creates a chronic disease.

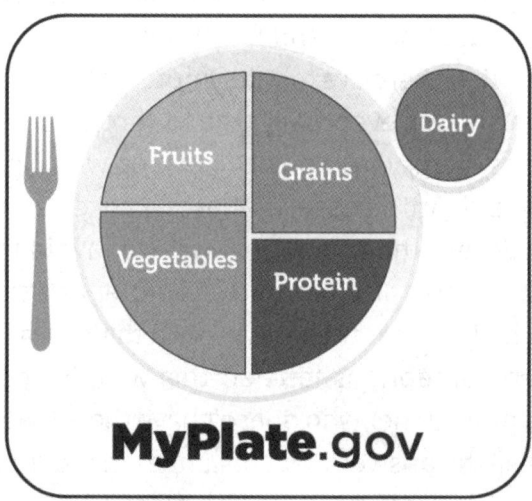

Figure: In-1 U.S. Government MyPlate guidelines

Recipe for Chronic Disease

In a large mixing bowl, combine processed grains, CAFO (Concentrated Animal Feeding Operations) meat, rancid vegetable oils, and ultra-pasteurized milk. Pour in a large amount of high-fructose corn syrup and sprinkle with electromagnetic fields (EMFs), chlorine, and fluoride. Bake while you sit at your computer. The end result is a chronic disease that will torture you for decades before you die.

What our government guidelines are telling us to eat is crazy.[1] If I wanted to create a diet plan for someone to gain weight and get sick, I would give them the standard American diet and have them eat every two to three hours.

Luckily, there are practitioners who are going against the grain. They take time with their patients, but insurance doesn't typically cover them because it's a lot more expensive to work this way, and patients don't need any drugs. Doctors who work outside the box are going to be held liable if they don't practice the conventional standard of care with their patients (even if they know it would be better for them not to), and the liability cost is very high—it could even mean their career is taken away from them.[2]

Let's take control and responsibility for getting our bodies what they need so that we can change the trajectory of our lives. I want to show you another way and give you the keys to unlock the door to preventing and reversing disease.

You can use the early signs of inflammation, such as joint pain, to allow you to see what needs to be worked on. Also, when you focus on avoiding chronic disease, you'll find your ideal weight as a side benefit, because fat is a symptom of a

---

[1] https://health.gov/our-work/nutrition-physical-activity/dietary-guidelines
[2] https://www.ncbi.nlm.nih.gov/pmc/articles/PMC3088386/

more significant health issue. We're also going to explore why your body is storing fat and creating inflammation in your joints, because understanding what is going on will point you toward opportunities for change.

I know you want to get to the root cause before something big hits you that could have been prevented. That's why you're reading this book—because on some level, you know there's more to it than just fate and genetics. Your life is not up to chance.

> Your life is not up to chance.

The first step is to look at the body as a whole system and not separate systems. We talk about hormones, muscles and bones, and the digestive system, but how often do you hear talk about how they interact? Looking at the body through this lens will give you a different perspective and help you see true, whole body health.

In Pilates, we talk a lot about whole body health and exercise the body as a whole, not just one muscle or joint at a time.[3] We also look at diet, hormones, and lifestyle choices to achieve true, whole body health.

---

[3] https://smile.amazon.com/Return-Life-Joseph-H-Pilates/dp/0976823209/ref=sr_1_8?crid=3RKS9112OLGO7&keywords=pilates+book&qid=1663281380&sprefix=pilates+book%2Caps%2C164&sr=8-8

Joe Pilates

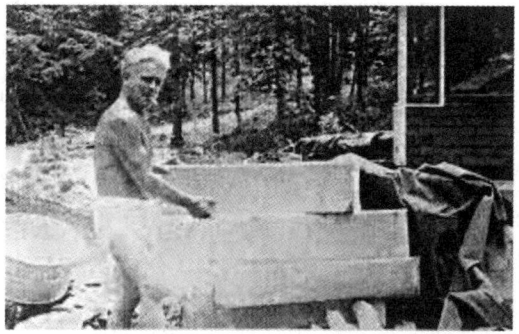

Figure In-2: Joe Pilates

Joseph Pilates was ahead of his time in his understanding of how movement could heal us from all sorts of physical ailments.[4] However, he did not understand the whole body health big picture. There's not much known about his eating habits, but there's been a lot said about his drinking and cigar smoking.

Throughout my journey with cancer, I realized that all the systems in the body are connected. They are *interdependent*, not independent. Until we fully understand and embrace this, we're going to keep spot treating our ailments, and we'll never achieve whole body health.

Since Joe was a boxer, I'm going to give you a one-two punch of looking at the whole body, instead of just muscles, joints, tendons, and ligaments. Of course, you need diet and exercise to shift how your body functions, but not necessarily in the way you think. We're going to talk about muscle

---

[4] https://smile.amazon.com/Return-Life-Joseph-H-Pilates/dp/0976823209/ref=sr_1_8?crid=3RKS9112OLGO7&keywords=pilates+book&qid=1663281380&sprefix=pilates+book%2Caps%2C164&sr=8-8

balancing and a low insulin diet to help you find your vibrance and maintain it for the rest of your life.

For example, if someone has recurring knee pain, they may go to different specialists and try to resolve it with different modalities—stem cells, physical therapy, Pilates, and so on—but they'll need both diet and muscle balancing to truly resolve their knee pain and keep it at bay. You've got to look at what is driving the inflammation in the knee from a root level, and this is going to be different for every person.

In this book, I'm going to give you a framework on what to look for in your body because we all need to know what our symptoms are telling us. I want you to feel empowered and in control of your health.

I'm going to give you tools so that you can work on resolving your own joint pain, losing unwanted weight, and preventing chronic disease. You can live freely with no fear of chronic disease. You are not a victim.

My publisher didn't want this book to be 700 pages long, so I couldn't fit everything in it, but I have even more information online, and below is a QR code to my website to help you access all of it for free. We also have a community of like-minded individuals who can answer your questions directly.

I am passionate about helping you take responsibility for your own health, and I want to get the tools you'll need into your hands.

Let's get started!

https://nutritionalpilates.com/step/book-resources-optin/

Chapter 1
Your Posture Hangs in the (Muscle) Balance

When I was in college, I was a dance major and doing the prerequisites for physical therapy school, but I was having back pain. It got to the point where I didn't enjoy dancing anymore because I was left aching so much afterward.

What in the world would I be like at forty-one if I hurt this much at twenty-one? I felt like the pain that I was experiencing was limiting my dreams and blocking my hopes for the future. How could I do physical therapy (PT) work if I couldn't even get through a dance class?

The physical therapy clinic where I was doing my internship was also working on my back. I was told the pain I was feeling was because of my scoliosis, which was so bad that the PTs called in other therapists to look at it.

After several months of treatment, nothing had really changed, and my left ankle had also started hurting. The PTs soon realized that my left arch had collapsed and had torqued my ankle, causing a twist in my pelvis, which then messed up my back.

It was my Pilates teacher who introduced me to the foot corrector apparatus and brought my attention to my muscle imbalances. By regaining my arch strength, I was able to untwist my pelvis, and today my scoliosis isn't visible. My back pain has never returned either, even through seven pregnancies. And here's the crazy part—within six months of starting Pilates, my right wrist (which had some tendinitis) also stopped hurting.

I realized that instead of looking at the one joint that was in pain (the current physical therapy model), you have to look at the whole body. An understanding of how each part of the body works together to inform the whole will give you tools that you can use to address your own health, no matter whether you are doing Pilates or some other form of movement.

So, What Is Pilates?

You may have seen Mari Windsor's mat Pilates videos or been to a Club Pilates franchise and done some reformer work. But what is it?

Pilates is a systematic approach to joint health and uses specific exercises and equipment to get your joints mobilized and stabilized so that there is balance around them.

The magic isn't those particular exercises or even the equipment—it's in the philosophy introduced by Joseph Pilates, who believed that his exercises should prepare us for our daily lives by training our bodies in a controlled environment for the wide variety of movements we may encounter.[5]

Chiropractors pop joints back into the right place, but this often means that they will pop out of place and require further adjustments. This happens because muscles attached to the joints pull them out of place. If you change the pull of those muscles, then you stabilize the joints and things not only stay in place but also track better. This is what we do in Pilates, which works beautifully alone or in synergy with other modalities, like chiropractic.

Pilates is about the quality of movement and alignment. More movement is not always better, because if you're doing something wrong, you're just training yourself to do it wrong more often, and that's not what we're going for. We want to train and correct our body mechanics and alignment in order to help those poor joints. I'd rather my clients did three reps well than twenty reps poorly.

Coming Back to the "Why"

We were active throughout the day before we invented modern conveniences that do the work for us, like washing machines, cars, and dishwashers. Today, we artificially put movement back into our lives with scheduled exercise.

Pilates is all about joint health. While exercise may help joints, it often does the opposite and can make them more imbalanced, depending on what we're doing—think of a runner with knee pain or a body builder who can't fully extend

---

[5] https://smile.amazon.com/Your-Health-Corrective-Exercising-Revolutionizes/dp/096149378X/ref=sr_1_1?crid=39KC62ONBPYVF&keywords=pilates+book+your+health&qid=1663282123&sprefix=pilates+book+your+health%2Caps%2C132&sr=8-1

their elbows. I tease my clients that, if they have a certain activity they want to do that is unhealthy for their joints, they need to do Pilates in order to compensate for it. For example, if they want to wear high heels, then they need to make sure they do their work in the studio. It's not that you can't do these things, you just have to know how what you're doing affects you and how to compensate for those actions.

Exercise will get the muscles pumping and the blood flowing, which is vital to getting nutrients, oxygen, and hydration to all the body's cells.[6] When blood circulates, it also takes out the trash via the lymphatic system. Good circulation is critical to detoxing the body, which is more important than ever in light of the massive toxin exposure that we are unable to avoid today.

Furthermore, exercise releases endorphins that literally help us feel better.[7] When we're depressed, we don't feel like exercising and would rather curl up in a ball in bed, but if we force ourselves to exercise, the endorphins will kick in. When they do, we'll be more likely to chase that feeling again, creating a positive spiral taking us toward better health.

It may startle you to read this, but you should NOT exercise to lose weight or to sculpt your body.

> You should NOT exercise to lose weight or to sculpt your body.

You may ask, "Why is the owner of a Pilates studio who trains fitness professionals saying this?"

Here's the dirty secret that no fitness professional wants to say out

---

[6] https://smile.amazon.com/Your-Health-Corrective-Exercising-Revolutionizes/dp/096149378X/ref=sr_1_1?crid=39KC62ONBPYVF&keywords=pilates+book+your+health&qid=1663282123&sprefix=pilates+book+your+health%2Caps%2C132&sr=8-1

[7] https://link.springer.com/article/10.2165/00007256-198401020-00004

loud—exercise will not make you lose weight alone, and spot treating an area of your body with it does not work.[8,9] Losing weight and looking better in your clothes are side benefits of exercise. This is to say nothing about long-term health and preventing chronic disease, but you've got to dig into what is truly causing inflammation and weight gain if you want the long-term results. You need to keep your eye on the prize and know that there's more than just exercise. It's never just exercise that is going to help someone transform their body, but it sure can help.

PILATES' LITTLE SECRET

Muscle balancing is the secret to Pilates. Every joint in your body has muscles on either side of it. In fact, there are multiple muscles on each side of your joints.

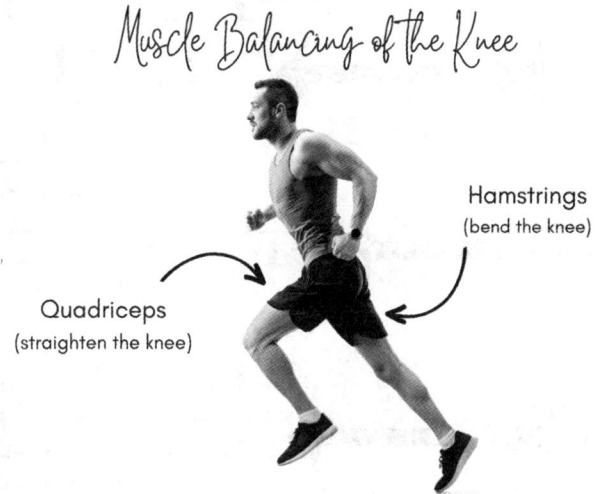

Figure 1-1: Muscle balancing of the knee

---

[8] https://www.sciencedirect.com/science/article/abs/pii/S0033062013001655
[9] https://www.sciencedirect.com/science/article/abs/pii/S0002822395003711

Let's take your knee, for example. You can straighten your knee (extension) or you can bend your knee (flexion). If you straighten your knee, the thigh muscles on the top (the quadriceps) create that movement. If you bend your knee, the muscles on the backs of your thighs (the hamstrings) do the work.

These two muscle groups work in opposition to each other, and both groups are composed of multiple muscles, or backup systems. It's never just one muscle that's moving while the others do nothing. When one is in motion (a concentric contraction), the other is lengthening (an eccentric contraction).

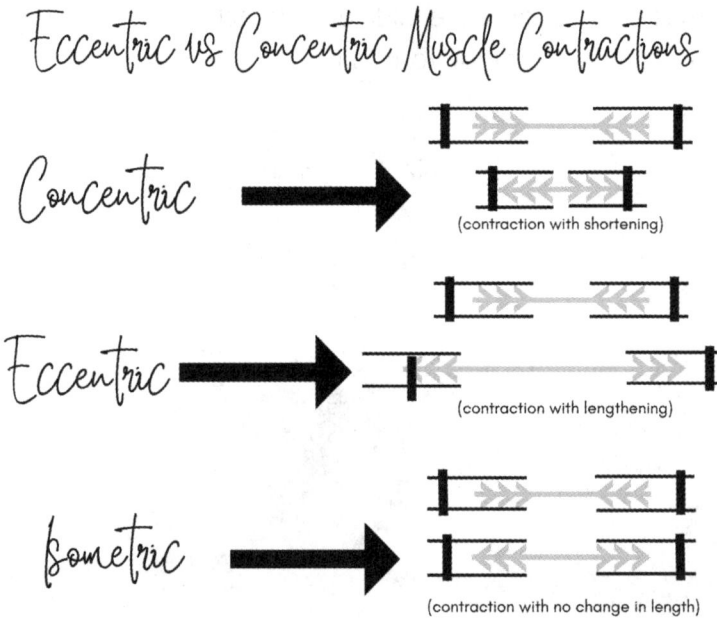

Figure 1-2: Eccentric versus concentric muscle contractions

When the muscles are not balanced, they pull the joint so that it doesn't track properly. This can cause inflammation and wear and tear on the joints. (The suffix "-itis" means inflammation.) When the joints aren't tracking well, there is inflammation, and you are ripe for injuries.

While you may want your quads to be stronger or look a certain way, that shouldn't be your only focus. I really want to drive this home because we often focus only on what I call *aesthetic sculpting*. When we want a certain body part to look a certain way and that's all we focus on, we end up with an injury or pain and wonder where that came from, as if it is totally unconnected.

Here's the silver lining—if you focus on the joints, you will actually get what your heart desires in terms of the aesthetic sculpting. But remember, it's a side benefit—the real goal is whole body health.

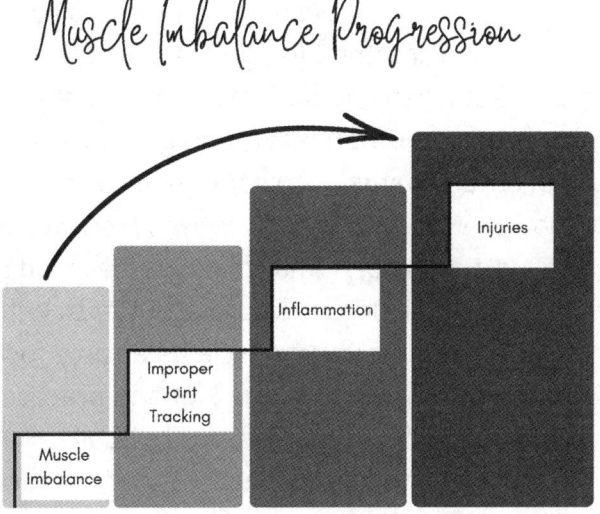

Figure 1-3: Sliding scale of muscle imbalances

So, how do we get there?

Muscle balancing is going to be different for every person, and that's why this book is not full of exercises. I'm tired of one-size-fits-all, quick-fix diets and exercise programs, aren't you? They don't work!

What you need are concepts and principles to help you customize your diet and workout. I believe this so intensely that my studio is called Personalized Pilates.

To attain this personalized experience, I'm going to give you the gold. If you understand the principle I'm about to share with you, you'll be able to customize any workout to your specific needs and pivot as time goes on to meet your new needs. So, here it is:

Do what you suck at.

> Do what you suck at.

Sounds silly and simplistic, doesn't it? Let me explain further.

If you are good at something, you're already likely balanced in that area. But when you hit a movement that you don't do well, that's when you should say, *I need to work on this.*

Human nature wants us to continually do the things that we are good at. We say to ourselves, *Hey, I rock at this exercise! I'm going to do it every day!* It may make us feel good because it strokes our ego, but it doesn't improve our muscle imbalance.

To effect change in your muscle balancing, focus on the exercises and movements you suck at and practice those as much as possible. This is what Pilates is actually all about—its exercises were created to help us see and work on muscle imbalance more easily.

You can use this principle in any modality. It doesn't matter if you're doing CrossFit, yoga, aerobics, or weightlifting. You just have to set your vanity and pride aside.

Does this mean that you can't do the other exercises that you know you're good at and like doing? No, but don't focus solely on those. Look at those exercises as the little treats to keep you going throughout the workout, so you don't just hate the whole thing and never want to come back.

If you choose exercise classes, I need to state the obvious—they won't be personalized (much) to you. You may have to do a few exercises on your own or separate from the class to fully "do what you suck at." This takes some serious self-discipline, and it's the main reason people may want to hire a professional with this philosophy—doing so allows them to not only have someone show them what they need to work on, but it also keeps them accountable.

Also, when taking classes, it's good to consider the instructor's goals and philosophy and compare them to your own. Choose wisely, because your time and your body matter.

Perfecting Your Posture

I define posture as how our bones are held in place when we're at rest. Understanding posture gives us significant clues as to what muscles are tight, loose, or weak and what we can do about correcting them.[10] But first we must know what ideal posture is and how our posture compares.[11] I have added diagrams to show you what body parts should be stacking up

---

[10] https://www.sciencedirect.com/science/article/abs/pii/S0002822395003711

[11] https://www.amazon.com/Muscles-Testing-Function-Posture-Kendall/dp/0781747805/ref=sr_1_1?gclid=Cj0KCQjwmouZBhDSARIsALYcoupL3i-UC5btrPdNfGggc5RWIK57UHb7lH6n-GGFIEwEJK0FJyctPxvgaAjFOEALw_wcB&hvadid=583842091583&hvdev=c&hvlocphy=9033834&hvnetw=g&hvqmt=e&hvrand=9019197448544091478&hvtargid=kwd-334009066524&hydadcr=22597_10356339&keywords=kendall+muscles+testing+and+function&qid=1663284037&s=books&sr=1-1

against each other (think of them like building blocks) from the front, the back, and the side, so that you can see what ideal posture should look like.

When looking at these drawings, please don't be too harsh on yourself if you don't line up perfectly. I can't stress enough that this is a journey, and these are tools that ensure we are headed in the right direction. Arriving at perfection is not the point. The point is to go toward perfection, but first you have to know what your goal is in order to do that.

I want you to look at your own posture. Take some selfies or have a friend take a photo of you from the front, side, and back and compare them to the diagrams to note the similarities and differences.

Front Posture Points

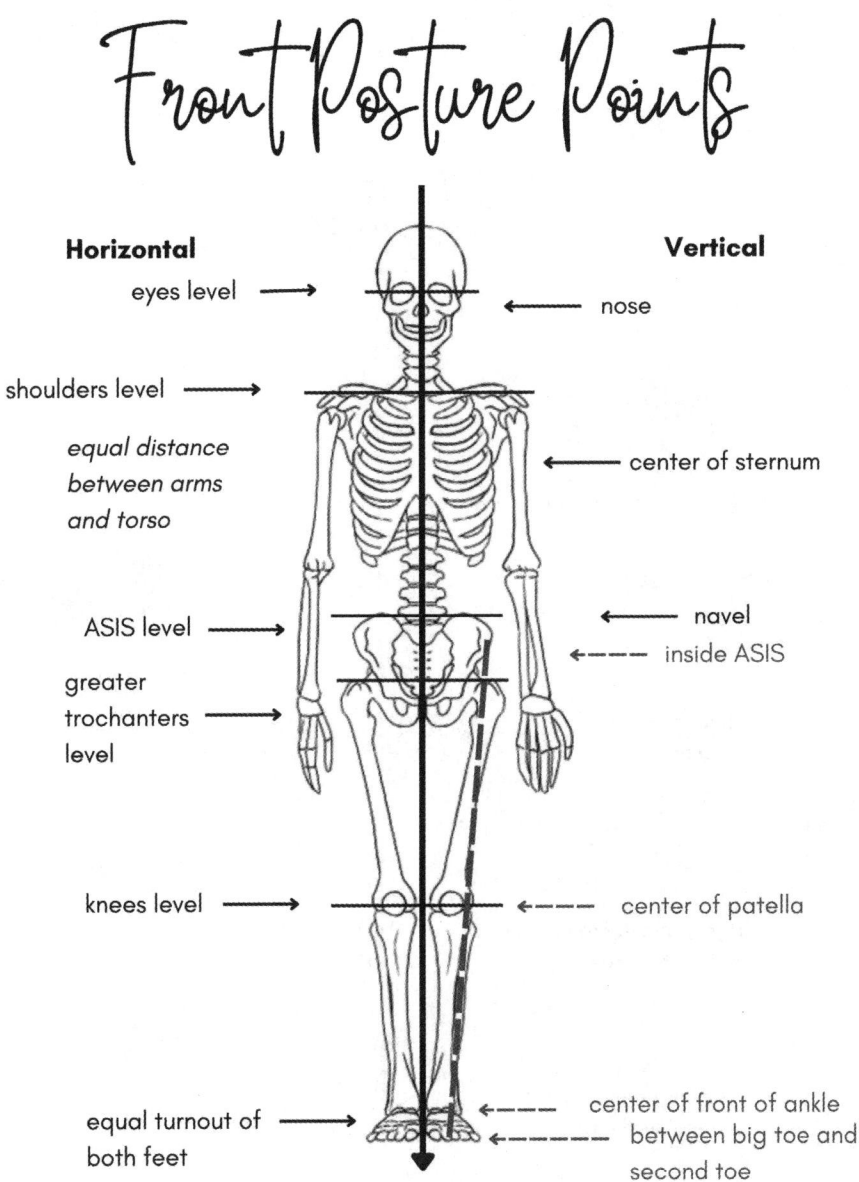

Figure 1-4: Front posture points

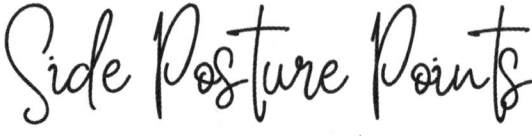

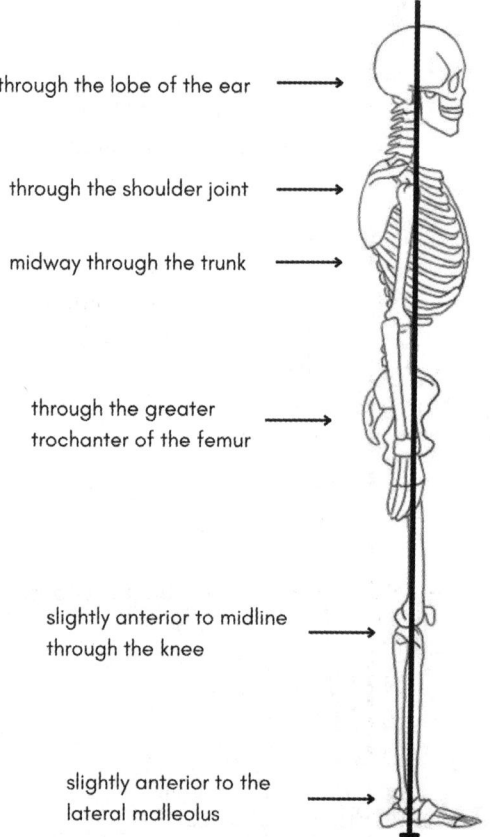

- through the lobe of the ear
- through the shoulder joint
- midway through the trunk
- through the greater trochanter of the femur
- slightly anterior to midline through the knee
- slightly anterior to the lateral malleolus

Figure 1-5: Side posture points

Back Posture Points

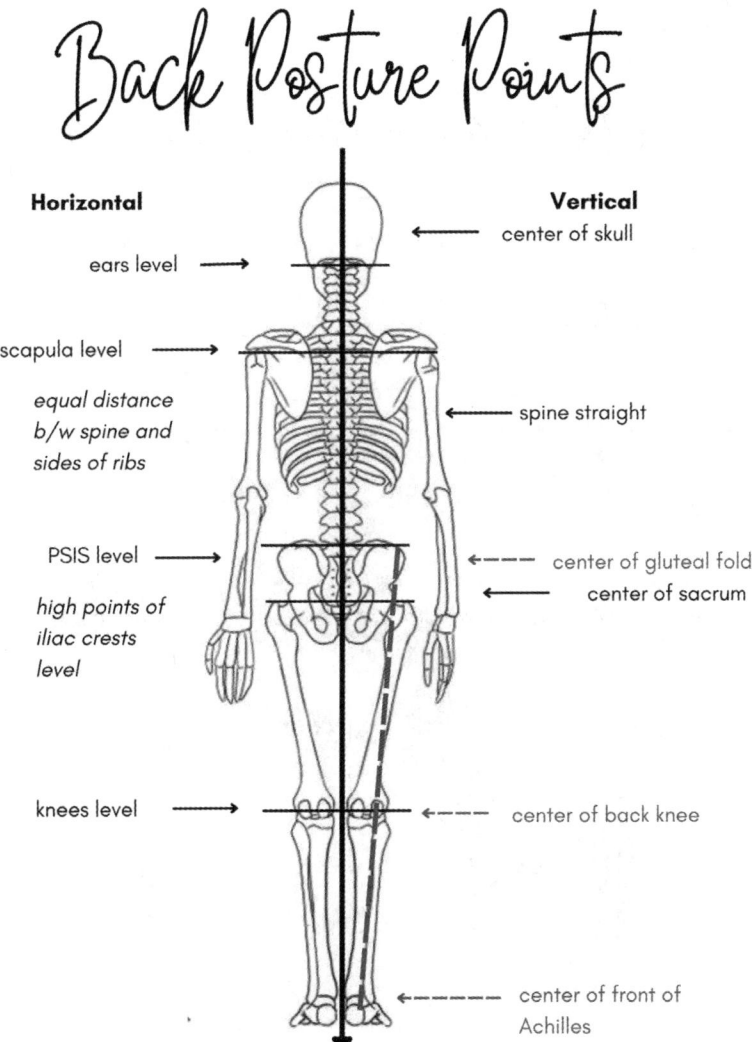

Figure 1-6: Back posture points

There are typical posture imbalances, or stereotypes, if you will. Seeing the list below will guide you toward knowing which muscle imbalances you may have. You can then compare the posture types with what you actually see and feel when you're moving.

Typical Imbalances with Common Posture Types

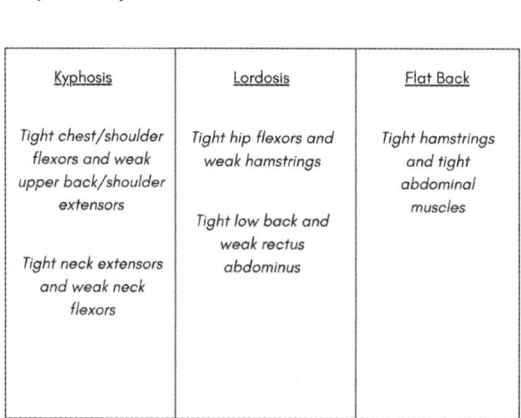

Kyphosis	Lordosis	Flat Back
Tight chest/shoulder flexors and weak upper back/shoulder extensors	Tight hip flexors and weak hamstrings	Tight hamstrings and tight abdominal muscles
Tight neck extensors and weak neck flexors	Tight low back and weak rectus abdominus	

Figure 1-7.a: Typical imbalances with common posture types

Posture Types

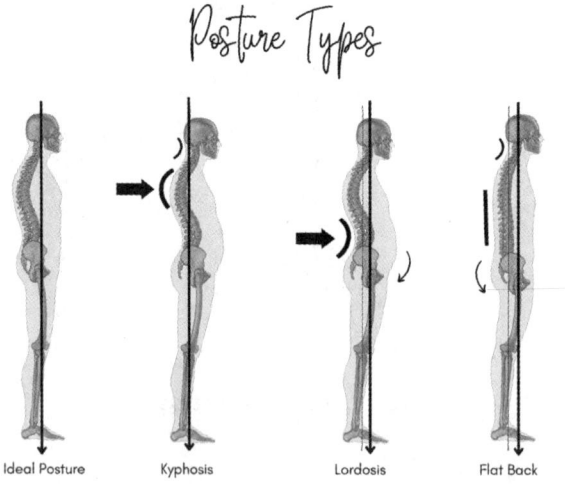

Figure 1-7.b: Typical imbalances with common posture types

Changing your posture is all about balancing your muscles—you want to lengthen what is tight and strengthen what is loose. Since all muscles are partnered with another that opposes them, we often see these imbalances affecting both sides of the joint, meaning one side is too tight and the other is too loose.

In Pilates, we work the muscles while they are creating movement (shortening) and while they are allowing movement (lengthening). While we "feel" what is shortening, we will also be working on the muscles that are lengthening. I call this *sneaky stretching*—you don't even notice that you are changing the resting length of the muscles so that you're more flexible. An example of this is the Teaser exercise where you feel your abdominals pulling you up, but you are also getting a sneaky stretch through the whole backside of your body, particularly the hamstrings. End result? Stronger abs and magically more flexible hamstrings.

Teaser

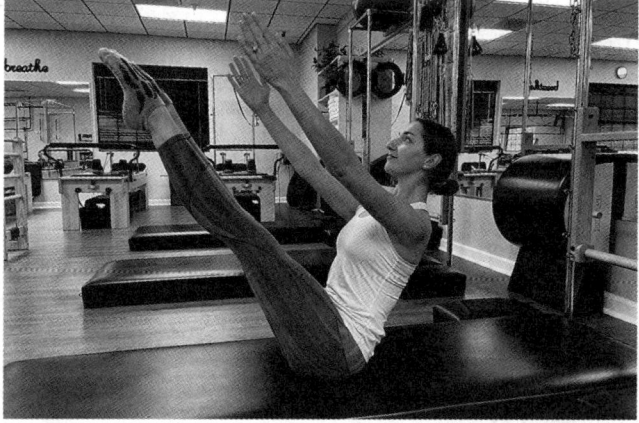

Figure 1-8: Teaser

I want to give you my quick and dirty fix for pretty much any posture. If you're sitting or standing, think of the crown of your head lifting and rising up and creating length, as if someone is grabbing you by a high ponytail and trying to pick you up (my ballet teacher used to literally do this.)

This is going to create length through your spine and actively decompress it; the other joints will magically fall into place, and your body will look more attractive. You can practice when you're standing in line for groceries, pumping gas, or sitting at your desk. As you continue to remind yourself to do this, you'll eventually do it on autopilot, and your weaker muscles will gradually get stronger as you hold this lengthened alignment. This was one of the techniques I used to retrain my posture. I still use it to this day, and now I'm passing it on to you so that you can find your length.

When I started seeing these concepts transform my body, I was so amazed that I enrolled in Pilates certification before I was even out of college. After just one semester, my transformation stunned my dance teachers.

It was revolutionary to finally have the control over my body that I had always wanted. I could do more turns with greater consistency, my flexibility was improved, and my leg extensions busted through previous walls. Not only did I move better, but I also lost inches all over. I was particularly fascinated by my thighs, which were stronger but had actually slimmed down.

I didn't have the bulging cheerleader look anymore, and I finally looked good in a bathing suit. The best part was that I had forgotten my back pain. I was hooked and knew that this paradigm was what I wanted to teach others.

Chapter 2
When You're Thrown Off Balance, Find YOUR Imbalances

You're probably wondering what your muscle imbalances are and what you need to work on, so I'm going to go through my top five and show you how to determine what you may be dealing with. (There is more info available online through the QR code at the end of the Introduction).

Before we get into it, I first want to tell you about Carrie. She was thirty-seven and about a year postpartum when she came to me and told me her shoulders felt tight and painful, and she often also had low back pain. While she was sitting, I gave her a wooden dowel to hold and asked her to bring it overhead. Right away, I knew she had some issues that we needed to work on.

Carrie held the bar very wide at its ends. Her elbows were bent, and she brought the bar up until it was about a foot in front of her face. Even in that position, the front of her ribs jutted forward, causing a huge arch in her lower back. This gave me indicators as to what we needed to work on, which is what we're going to dive into next.

THE TOP FIVE MUSCLE IMBALANCES

When looking at this list, you'll need to adjust according to what is going on for you specifically and your current fitness level. There are a host of other imbalances, but I see the following five more than most others.

1. Tight lats

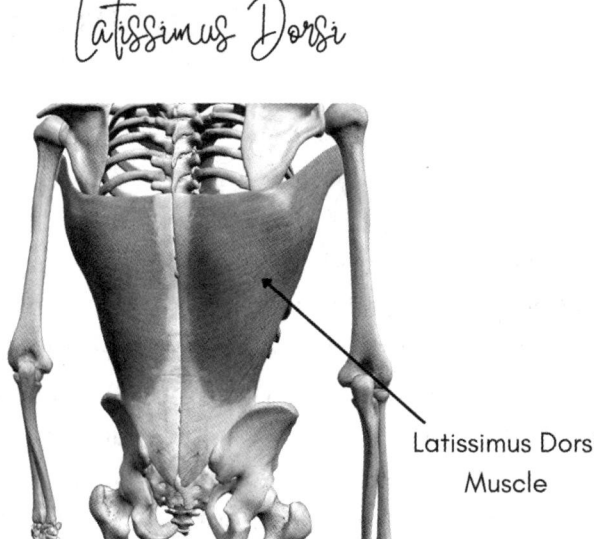

Figure 2-1: Lats anatomy

"Lats" is short for *latissimus dorsi*, a muscle running from the top front of your upper arm bone, under your armpit, to your lower back and sacrum area. It's a long muscle with many nuanced functions, including internally rotating the arm bone and rolling the shoulder forward.

The easy way to see if this is an issue for you is to lie down on a mat with your knees bent and feet flat to take any pressure off your lower back. With your arms down by your hips, check if your bra hook is touching the mat (lower/

mid ribs). You want it down on the mat. Now, take your arms from beside your hips and bring them straight up toward the ceiling, parallel to each other. Bring your arms overhead to see how far you can go without losing contact between the floor and your bra hook. (Bizarrely enough, everyone seems to know where their bra hook would be, even if they don't wear one.)

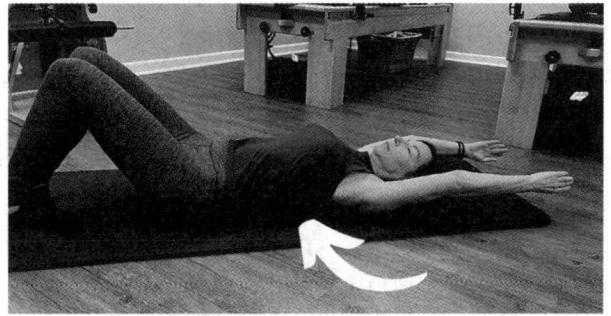

Watch that the bra hook doesn't come off the floor when the arms go overhead

Figure 2-2: Ribcage Arms

Can your arms reach the floor overhead? If you can, does your bra hook pop off the ground? If you can't touch the floor with your bra hook down, this is a good indicator that your lats are tight. In Pilates, we call this Ribcage Arms. This could be an exercise in and of itself, or we can use it as an assessment. I used this as a postpartum exercise because I get very tight in my lats when I'm pregnant, but now I use it more as a warmup.

To open your lats, you want to make sure that you keep your ribcage still when you're doing arm work. Not that moving your ribcage is bad, but if you don't hold it still, you won't stretch your lats. If you lay a resistance band out and pull one end, it doesn't actually stretch—it just moves. You have to hold the opposite end still to stretch it. And that's where holding the ribcage still is helping to stretch the lats.

If your bra hook came off the floor, that's a sign that your lats are saying, "We're done. We can't go any further." That's the point when you have to humble yourself and stop, or you'll lose the stretch. Most people can't get their arms to touch the ground behind them with their ribcage neutral, which is why tight lats is on this list.

In Pilates, we have exercises to help open up the lats, such as the Lat Cat, the Elephant, the Short Box, the Flat Back, the Mermaid, and so on. Here's the key that no one talks about, however—most of the time when people are engaged in these exercises, they're not focusing on their lats opening, and they do things like bend their arms or not bring their arms all the way overhead. Opening their lats can enhance the whole exercise, and through this, they can really get to the depth of this muscle imbalance.

2. Weak serratus anterior (pronounced "sir-a-tus" anterior)

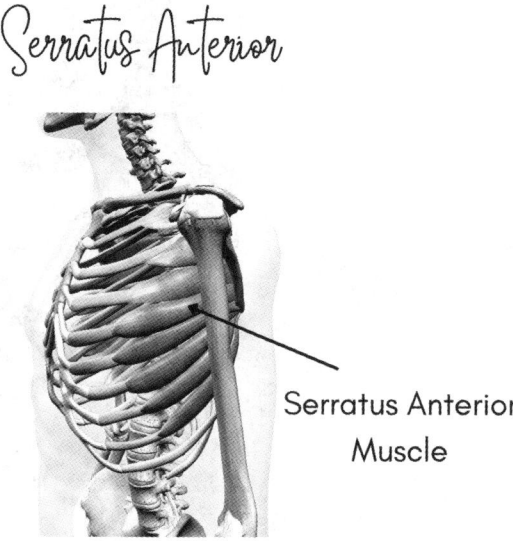

Figure 2-3: Serratus Anterior anatomy

This is a muscle that no one ever talks about because you can't see it, so aesthetically, it's worthless. However, I believe ignoring this muscle is one of the key factors in developing rotator cuff issues.

The serratus anterior attaches on the inside edge of the scapula (shoulder blade) and wraps around the ribcage through the armpit while underneath the shoulder blade.

One of its jobs is to help you upwardly rotate your shoulder blades. If you bring your arms overhead, do your shoulder blades come up and are they lifted high? Can you bring your shoulder blades back down? If not, that's usually a sign of a weak serratus anterior.

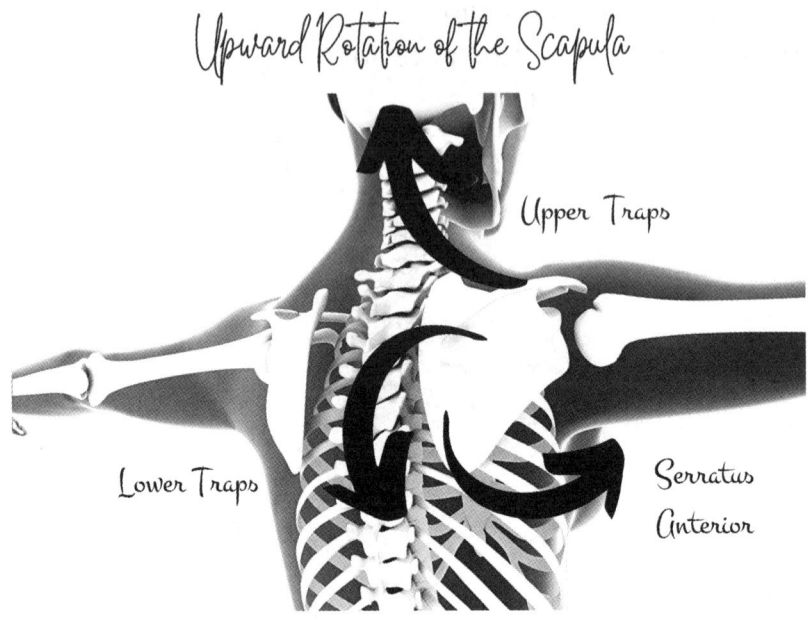

Figure 2-4: Upward rotation

There are three muscles that create a pivot for the shoulder blade to rotate on its axis. If one of these isn't working, then the whole shoulder blade doesn't spin on its axis like it's supposed to and instead shifts toward the other two. In this case, the shoulder blade spins up when the serratus anterior is out to lunch and the arms are overhead. We may say things like "Keep your shoulders down," but if the serratus anterior is weak, that's just really not going to happen.

Arms Overhead

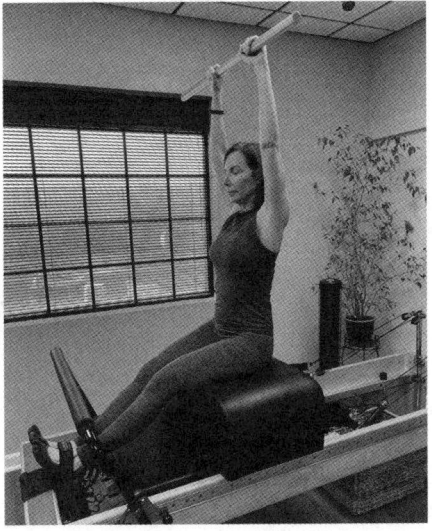

Shoulders should be down – Serratus Anterior

Figure 2-5: Arms overhead with shoulders up

There's another way to check if you have a weak serratus anterior—have a friend take a picture of you from the top looking down when you're doing a plank or a push-up to see if the inside edge of your shoulder blade is lifting up off your ribcage. If so, that's a sign your serratus anterior is not doing its job to suction the shoulder blade down onto the ribcage (this is a form of protraction).

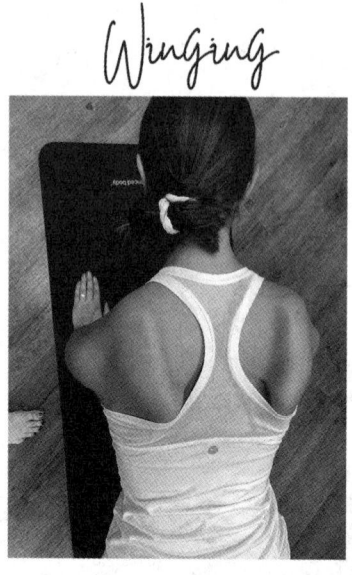

Winging

Inside edges of shoulder blades should lie flat on the back — Serratus Anterior

Figure 2-6: Winging push-up

To balance this, get in a quadruped position (i.e., on all fours). Keep your elbows straight and bring your shoulder blades together. (This isn't the serratus anterior but the opposing muscles, which will allow you to feel the serratus better.) Separate your shoulder blades as wide as possible to turn the serratus on. Be aware of other "cheat" movements, such as your shoulders coming up to your ears, your elbows bending, or your back bending or arching. You want to bring the whole torso up between the shoulder blades past where you would stay in neutral for a plank/push-up. That's where the serratus anterior works really hard, and this is what you want to practice. Here, the assessment is the exercise.

Sternum Drops

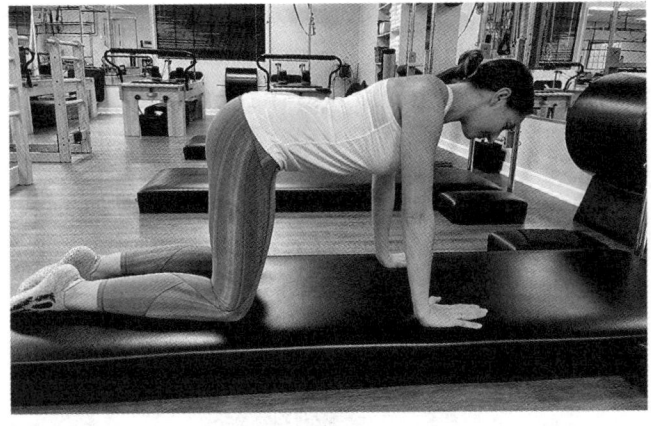

Bring the shoulder blades together with straight arms and back

Figure 2-7: Sternum drops

Elephant

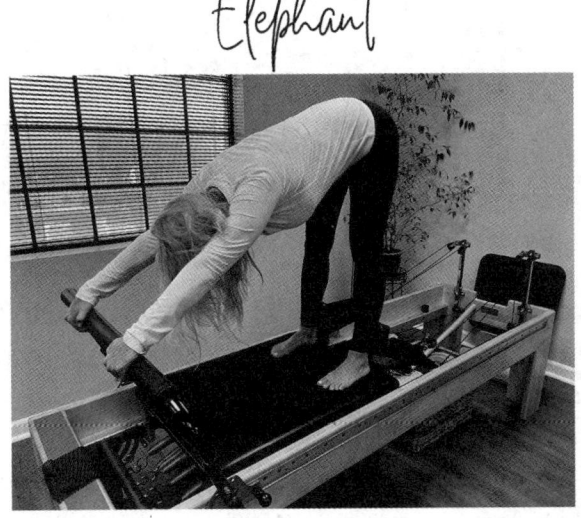

Hands shoulder width apart, straight arms, pull the bar apart

Figure 2-8: Elephant

In Pilates, we also do things like planks; here, the serratus strength is foundational. You can also work on this when you're in the Elephant (see Figure 2-8) or using a wooden dowel on the Short Box by pulling the bar/footbar wider without bending your elbows, which is going to cause the serratus anterior to fire. This will be very difficult and makes most people shake.

3. Tight pecs

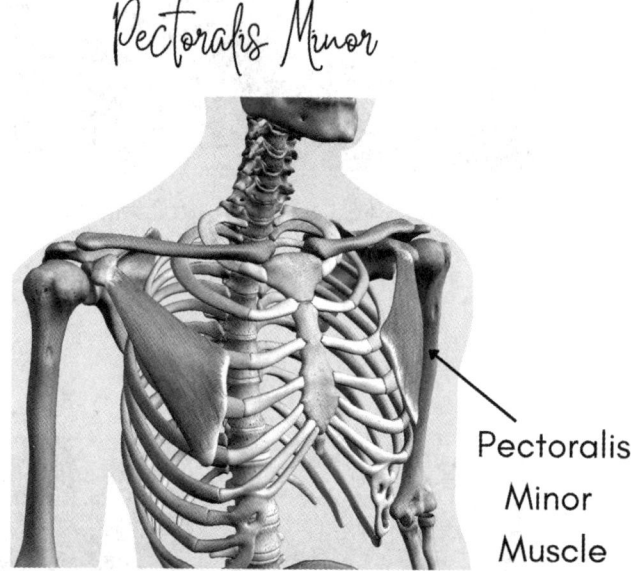

Figure 2-9: Pecs anatomy

The pectoralis major and minor cause your shoulders to roll forward and your chest to close up in a subtly different way than the lats do. People talk about this a lot—it is so common today with all our computer time.

Sitting up tall (as we talked about in the last chapter) is incredibly helpful to opening the front of the chest up, but we're going to take it a step farther. I want you to feel where your shoulders actually should be in a neutral position, so go ahead and try this. The weirder it feels and the more foreign it is, the tighter and more "off" you are.

Neutral Shoulders

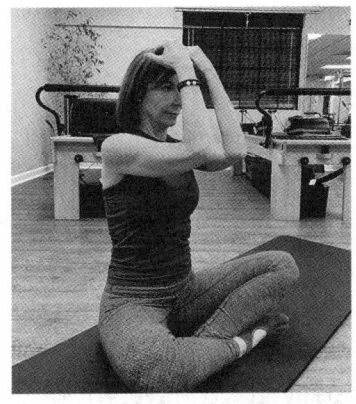
1. Hands on head, elbows forward

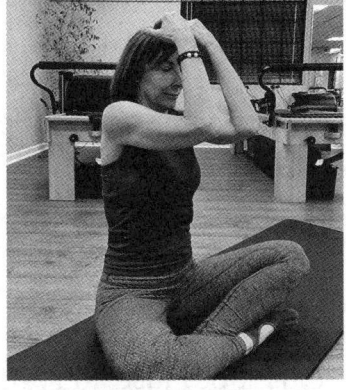
2. Lift shoulders up

Figure 2-10.a: Neutral shoulders

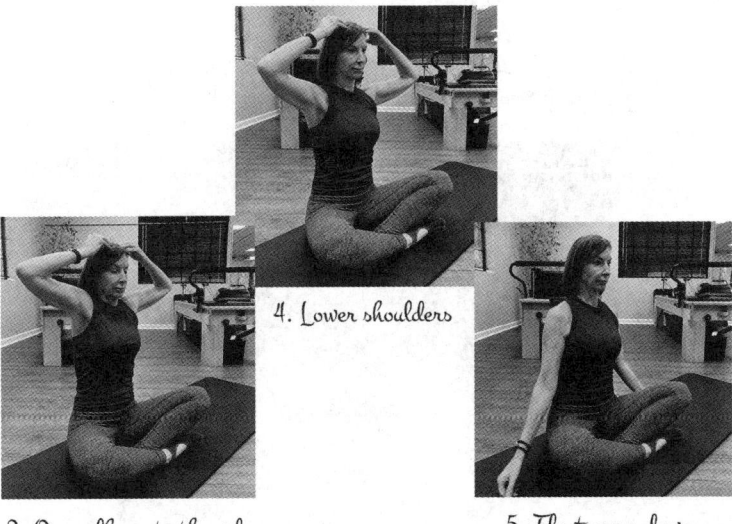

3. Open elbows to the side

4. Lower shoulders

5. Float arms down without moving shoulders

Figure 2-10.b: Neutral shoulders

Start by putting both your hands on top of your head. With your elbows pointing forward, lift your shoulders up, open your elbows out to the side and keep them there while you drop your shoulders down. Keep your shoulders where they are and slowly let your arms drift down to your sides. This is your neutral shoulder position and where you should lie, ideally.

Did it feel weird? If it did, let's make sure that we open up the front of the chest. This is a quick reset that you can do as a way to recalibrate your posture during a long, hard day wherever you are.

Another way to check this area is by lying on your back on a semi-hard surface with your knees bent and feet flat. Do the backs of your shoulders touch the floor, or are they lifted up off the floor? If they are lifted, it is a good indicator that you're tight because you've actually got the weight of your body trying to open your chest up in this position—your pecs are so tight that they're not even allowing your chest to open up when you have that help.

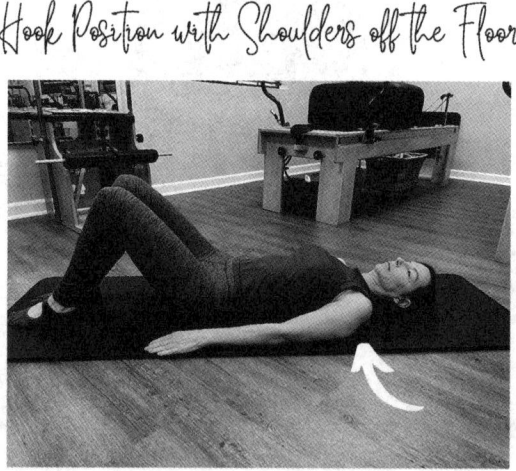

Shoulders and palms pressing into the mat

Figure 2-11: Hook position with shoulders off the floor

In Pilates, exercises like Hug a Tree, Press Backs, and Chest Expansion are some that actively work the pecs while they're in a stretched position. That way, we're working on the eccentric contraction and resetting the resting length so that they stay open.

4. Tight psoas (pronounced "so-az")

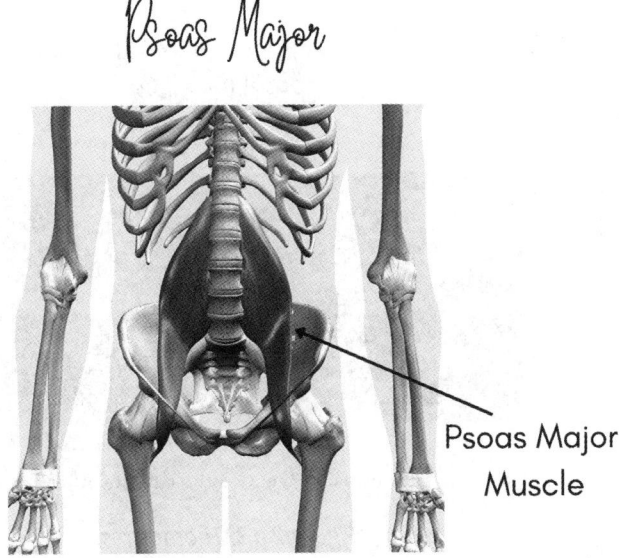

Figure 2-12: Psoas anatomy

This is another muscle that you may or may not have heard of because it runs deep along the front of your spine, behind your organs, and all the way down into the inside top of your thigh bone. In other words, no one can see it. However, there's a huge amount of dysfunction and discussion about it because we sit so much in the modern age. (In fact, you've probably heard experts say, "Sitting is the new smoking.")

The easiest way to address a tight psoas is to not sit all day, every day. Stand up and move around, if at all possible.

This may be something you need to work up to, so don't throw your desk out too quickly.

Here's how you can check your psoas and monitor your progress. Lie on your back and bring both knees to your chest so you can feel your thighs against your chest. Now, hold on under one knee and lengthen the thigh on the opposite side out toward the ground to see how far you can go without letting the knee that's in by your chest move away from it.

Thomas Test

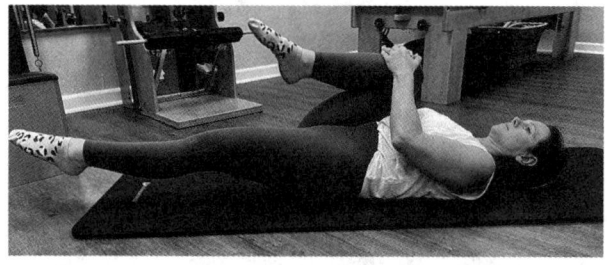

Hold one knee in while lengthening out the other leg — Psoas

Figure 2-13: Thomas test

Often, when people do this, they have a very difficult time getting their lengthened leg all the way on the ground without the other leg moving—that's what we want to work on. Since you have a right and left psoas, you can check both. You may be asymmetrical; this usually occurs due to scoliosis or lifestyle habits, so keep your eye out for asymmetry in the way you carry things or perform other tasks.

One of the easiest ways to open up the psoas besides getting more upright movement in daily life is to perform exercises with hip extension, which means opening up the front of the hips in an active way. Exercises like Prone Hip Extension, Swimming, Single and Double Leg Kicks, Bridging, and Swan are examples from Pilates, but anything working the hamstrings/glutes to open the front of the hip is great for this, as it will require the psoas to eccentrically open.

5. Tight back extensors

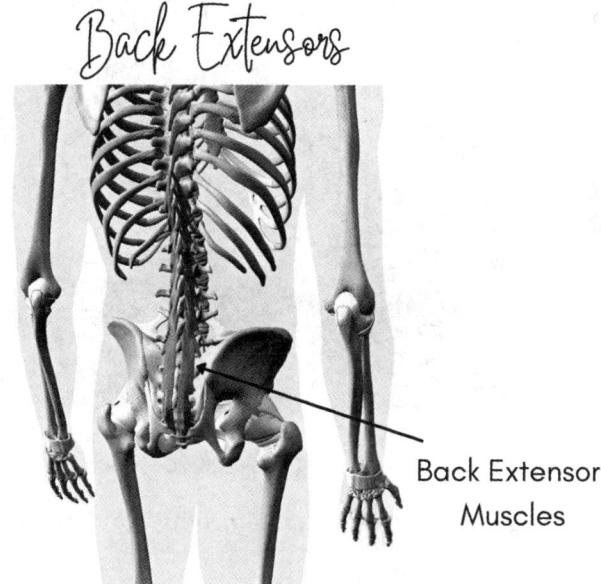

Figure 2-14: Back extensors anatomy

Most people feel it if their low back muscles are on what I call "permanent lockdown" because they will commonly have an achy low back at the end of the day. This is because those low back muscles can't contract anymore and never release. What we need is to release them and give them different options.

If you aren't sure, you can check this by lying on your back with your knees bent and feet flat. I'm going to have you do what we call in Pilates the Pelvic Clock, but we're just going to do part of it. I want you to tip your pelvis to get your waistband to touch the floor and then tip it the other way to get it to come off the floor. Go back and forth and note what touches and what doesn't. Those who have a really tight low back can't get it on the floor—they may even say it isn't possible.

Pelvic Clock – Neutral

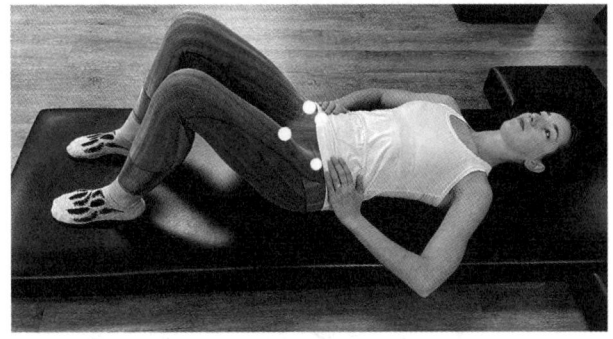

Hip bones (ASIS) and pubic bone in the same plane

Figure 2-15.a: Pelvic clock – neutral, 6 o'clock, and 12 o'clock

Pelvic Clock – 12 o'clock
(Anterior Tilt)

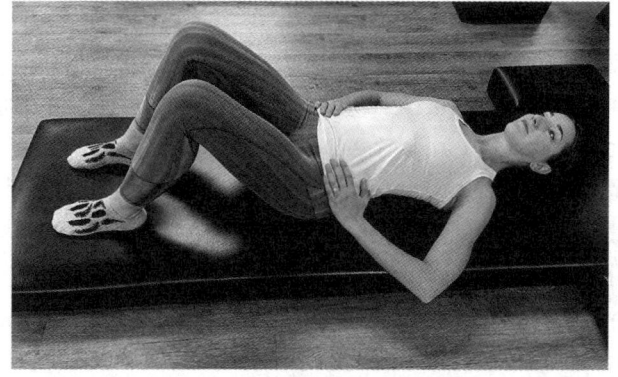

Arched back – waist off the mat as high as possible

Figure 2-15.b: Pelvic clock – neutral, 6 o'clock, and 12 o'clock

Pelvic Clock – 6 o'clock
(Posterior Tilt)

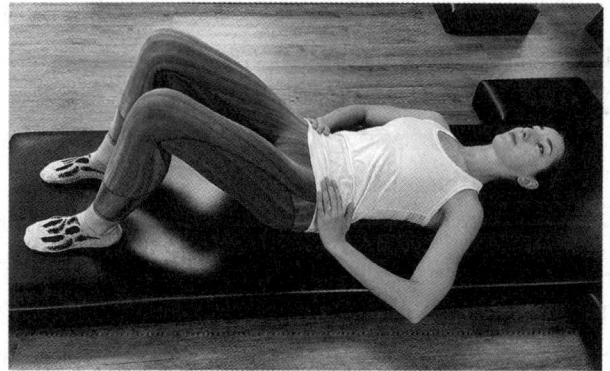

Tucked under bum – waist on the mat

Figure 2-15.c: Pelvic clock – neutral, 6 o'clock, and 12 o'clock

Spinal motion is fundamental to Pilates, which is why there are so many exercises incorporating it. In fact, we now know that you need this to get nutrients to and remove wastes from the spinal discs, as they don't have their own blood supply.

You can actually revitalize your discs and prevent issues by making sure you get your spine moving and articulating.[12] This particular movement is focused on just the lumbar (or lower) back, and I call it the Deep Posterior Tilt. This is where you tuck the pelvis under so that the low back touches the floor. This happens not from the glutes (butt cheeks) clenching but from your rectus abdominis (six-pack muscle).

The rectus abdominis attaches at your pubic bone and goes up to your sternum (breastbone). It pulls your pubic bone toward your chin and opposes the low back extensors. Exercises that "get your abs" will open up the back if they are utilizing the deep posterior tilt.

If you have tightness here, you may notice that exercises where you use the deep posterior tilt just don't seem to go well—in fact, you suck at them. Rolling Like a Ball usually goes down in a thump. Roll Up has your legs popping up in the air. In Rollover, you just can't get your butt off the mat without using your hands.

Does any of this sound familiar? These kinds of exercises really highlight this imbalance in a very obvious way, so work on them in a modified fashion as you build up your strength and range of motion. Doing the Pelvic Clock from the assessment is very therapeutic and will help to release those low back muscles quite a bit. This is a very common issue, which is why there are so many Pilates exercises that spotlight it.

---

[12] http://dx.doi.org/%2010.24966/PMRD-8670/100022

Spotting Additional Balance Issues

If you did not find that any of these issues were yours, I want to let you know that there are a lot of other imbalances. These are just what I consider the most common. Some other common imbalances include things like a weak core (this is talked about extensively nowadays, which I'm so excited to see), weak shoulder extensors, weak/tight hamstrings, weak inner thighs, weak abdominals, weak ankle dorsi flexors, and weak wrist flexors. These are the areas that I see clients struggling with the most when they come to see me, but again, you may have your own unique thing going on.

Keep in mind that as you age and experience life, these imbalances are going to shift—you may have a baby, you may be in a car accident, you may have a poor workstation, or you may have some other life change. The muscle imbalances reflect how you're using your body. If you change how you use your body, you're going to change those muscle imbalances, for the good or bad.

Is There Such a Thing as "Good" Pain?

Whether you're working out or moving around in daily life, it's important to know and understand that pain is your friend. This may sound odd, so let me give you an example.

One of my clients, Pam, had a lot of joint pain. Every time I asked how she was feeling, she told me she was in pain. It took me a bit to realize that she was describing hurting, stretching, and working as "pain." We had to delve into the semantics

> Pain is your friend. This may sound odd, so let me give you an example.

in her words to determine what exactly was actually causing her real pain and what wasn't.

Pain is our body's way of saying, "Hey, this is not good for me. Please stop."[13] Our bodies are designed to give us feedback. However, today we often ignore or override it and say things like "No pain, no gain."

But that's not what we should be doing—we should listen to our bodies, connect with what we're feeling, and make the appropriate choice about how to proceed. If something truly hurts and causes pain, that's when you need to back off. Getting the message "that's not right for me right now" is a blessing and means that you may need to modify an exercise to make it easier for the time being. A great Pilates teacher, Michelle Larson, often says that we are already good at pain so we don't need to practice it. She means that our bodies can already do a movement with poor mechanics that create pain, so let's choose something different in order to get a different outcome.

This takes a lot of humility because it is hard to back off, especially in front of others. We're very much a society that praises accomplishments: *I did this; therefore, I'm a good person.* But if we want to get out of pain, that's not what we want to focus on.

It's not just about hitting the number of reps or going all the way just for the sake of achievement or looking good—it's about focusing on quality instead. Remember, the root issue is muscle imbalances, and if our body is screaming "This hurts!" we're actually making the imbalances worse. So, do what is truly better for your body in the long run by listening to it and respecting it.

---

[13] https://doi.org/10.1073/pnas.0408576102

My vision is to empower and educate others so that they can discern what their body's specific needs are and how to adjust when things shift over time. That is true health—not only being in shape but also knowing how to nurture your body. At the end of the day, you're the one that has to live in it.

THREE STEPS TO BALANCING MUSCLE IMBALANCES

Here are the three steps I suggest for correcting muscle imbalances so that you can become that person who takes responsibility for their own body.

1. Know what ideal is

We already talked about perfect alignment, but when going a little deeper into whatever exercise you're doing—whether it's Pilates, strength training, or yoga—ask yourself: *What is correct alignment for this exercise/activity? Where does your foot go? What is your pelvis doing? What is the ideal way to do it?*

If you don't know what perfection is, how in the world are you going to be able to go toward attaining it?

2. Know what you suck at

This is another way of saying you should know your muscle imbalances and what you're working on. I quiz my Pilates teacher training students on this all the time—they are responsible for knowing this about every client they work with, and you should know this about yourself like the back of your hand. If you don't, how can you address your issues?

If you don't know what your current muscle imbalances are, a good instructor is worth their weight in gold in terms of assessing what's going on and giving you the appropriate exercises to address it. They should also educate you on whatever exercise they take you through (and you should relish in this education!)

An instructor should say things like "Try to get your shoulders down" or "Do you see that your shoulders are up?" Some might take it further and say, "When your shoulders are up, that's telling me your serratus is not working optimally, so we'll work on that," and connect you to the exercises that will help you. Ultimately, this will allow you to know your body better.

3. Know how to improve what you suck at
This step includes choosing the exercises that will challenge you in your muscle imbalances and having good form in whatever you do. This is where humility comes in and where you may not want to keep up with your friends or everyone else in class if you aren't able to do something without pain or good form.

You may need to alter your timing to go slower or faster or change the resistance level on springs or weights to make it more appropriate to what you can do. You may need to change your range of motion by making the exercise smaller or bigger so that you can do it correctly, or you may need to change the type of exercise you're doing based on how your body responds.

At the time of this writing, I am postpartum from my seventh child. Throughout my pregnancy, my low back and psoas have gotten tighter because my pelvis has been supporting a ten-pound baby. I am working on my deep posterior tilt quite a bit (I don't have a diastasis recti—an abdominal separation from pregnancy that would indicate not to do spinal flexion)[14,15,16,17,18] and boy, do I suck at exercises focused on this! My lats and pecs were crazy tight after this last pregnancy in particular. They have opened up, but I continue to work on that.

Additionally, I need to work on my forearm strength, inner thigh flexibility, and deltoid strength, so I make sure to incorporate exercises focusing on these areas into my workouts. What I do has to be intentional because if I just rely on doing a workout, I will magically "forget" all the things that are so hard!

Each person is a little different, but I have found that if I exercise a hard thirty to forty-five minutes every other day, I get the maximum strength- and flexibility-building results. If I work out every day, my body doesn't have enough time to recuperate, and I just don't have a fulfilling workout.

On alternate days, I take a nice hike or engage in another kind of activity in nature that's more focused on cardio. That's what works for me right now. Hopefully, it helps you see that you can create workouts that are targeted, enjoyable, and effective based on what your body tells you.

A LITTLE ABOUT CARDIOVASCULAR EXERCISE

Remember that cardio is going to increase circulation, which allows you to get nutrients to your cells and get the waste

---

[14] https://www.ncbi.nlm.nih.gov/pmc/articles/PMC6454249/
[15] https://journals.lww.com/jwhpt/Abstract/2014/05000/Progressive_Therapeutic_Exercise_Program_for.3.aspx
[16] https://journals.viamedica.pl/ginekologia_polska/article/view/56088
[17] https://www.ncbi.nlm.nih.gov/pmc/articles/PMC8136546/
[18] https://smile.amazon.com/Diastasis-Recti-Solution-Abdominal-Separation/dp/098965396X/ref=sr_1_4?crid=3JG68TFKSJQWR&keywords=katie+bowman+books&qid=1663772537&sprefix=katie+bowman+books%2Caps%2C153&sr=8-4

out. We can easily achieve a beautiful cardio interval training effect in higher levels of Pilates workouts, but you never hear people mention this because that's not the point of Pilates.

We want to focus on getting good mechanics as a priority, which, for most people, means they have to go slower at first, and as a result, they do not have as much of a cardio workout. They will still get circulation benefits but not so much a heart pumping kind of thing. To incorporate cardio while you're improving at muscle balancing, take brisk walks, hikes, or jogs so that you're not compromising form, but you're still getting your heart going.

One quick note here—a lot of people use a treadmill, perhaps because they are in a city or it's wintertime. A treadmill can actually create some hip dysfunction. You're not using hip extensors to push off while on a conveyor belt because it moves for you and alters your gait dynamics.[19] No matter what cardio (or everyday) activities you do, make sure they aren't working against you in balancing your muscles. Paying attention to these imbalances may be able to save you some work by minimizing or shifting those choices.

As Pam and Carrie worked on their imbalances, they not only regained function and relieved pain, but they also became more in tune with their bodies and learned how to take care of them going forward.

This meant that, as her child got bigger and heavier, she could still play with her, allowing Carrie to be a fun mom. She now understands where her Achilles heel is so that she can be proactive in preventing back and shoulder pain in future

---

[19] https://smile.amazon.com/Move-Your-DNA-Movement-Expanded-ebook/dp/B0718X8N7H/ref=sr_1_1?crid=3JG68TFKSJQWR&keywords=katie+bowman+books&qid=1663772537&sprefix=katie+bowman+books%2Caps%2C153&sr=8-1

pregnancies, which are no longer scary since she knows how to take care of her body.

Pam learned to differentiate hard movement from painful movement, which allowed her to push herself in an appropriate way without injury. This understanding took away her fear of movement because she now knows how to read her body and protect her joints.

Exercise is all about joint health. Pilates, cardio, weight-lifting, yoga, you name it—they won't help you lose fat. But if they don't help you lose weight, what does?

Chapter 3
The Surprising Effects of Insulin

Andrea came to me frustrated and with very little hope. She was forty-seven and was doing "all the right things." She had been working at reducing calories and increasing exercise, but to no avail. She had tried many different diet and exercise programs, but none had worked for her. Sure, she had lost some weight, but she gained it back as soon as she finished a program.

Andrea wanted to understand what was going on with her body, and why she was so "broken." What I explained opened her eyes to understanding how her body worked.

I suggested we shift her diet by taking into account her individual needs, and the weight slid gradually and effortlessly from her. Once she was at her ideal weight, we transitioned her to a maintenance program, and she's kept the weight off since. This process gave her renewed hope and an understanding of how to take care of her body so that she feels like she can be successful in going forward into the next phase of her life. She feels sexy and vibrant again. The only problem was that she had to buy new clothes!

Everything We've Been Taught About Dieting Is Wrong

Andrea had been taught that calories in have to be equal to or less than calories out in order to lose weight—but this a flat-out lie. There is no evidence supporting this idea, and it has been shown unequivocally to not produce the results desired over and over again.[20,21,22,23] I'm sure that you already know this from your own experience, yet many health professionals and government agencies continue to support and promote this concept.

Focusing on calories does not take hormones and other key influential factors into account when determining how much you weigh and how healthy you are. Food quality, the time you take your meals, macronutrients (protein, carbohydrates, and fats), bio-individuality, environmental toxins, epigenetics, digestion, hormones, stress, and many other things can drastically affect how you process the food that you eat.[24,25,26]

My goal is to give you the tools that allow you to understand the bigger picture, then create a personalized plan for you. Every one of us is different— there is no one-size-fits-all diet, no matter what a salesperson tells you. However, an understanding of some basic biological processes will give you the framework to create a plan for yourself.

---

[20] https://journals.physiology.org/doi/full/10.1152/ajpendo.00156.2017
[21] https://jamanetwork.com/journals/jamainternalmedicine/article-abstract/2686146
[22] https://doi.org/10.1016/j.ehb.2014.04.002
[23] https://academic.oup.com/ajcn/article/115/5/1243/6522166
[24] https://onlinelibrary.wiley.com/doi/abs/10.1111/obr.12603
[25] https://www.sciencedirect.com/science/article/abs/pii/S0002822307014794
[26] https://journals.physiology.org/doi/full/10.1152/ajpgi.00285.2004

I want to introduce you to an amazing researcher named Dr. Weston A. Price. He was a dentist who was frustrated with the increase in tooth decay that he saw in his practice over the years. He was determined to find out if there were any truly healthy cultures in the world and, if so, what they were doing that we weren't.

Price traveled the world over the next decade, visiting remote regions where people were eating native foods, preparing them as they had for thousands of years. What he found was truly astonishing—all of them had ten times the amount of fat-soluble vitamins in their diets compared to ours.[27] (Keep in mind that this was back in the 1930s—the standard American diet has gone further downhill since then.)

I dismissed the fact that Price didn't focus on this and instead focused on the native tribes not eating the "foods of modern civilization." That didn't make any sense to me, but the more nutrient-dense aspect of his findings did. However, it took me years to really figure out what he saw from the beginning.

What Insulin Does to Our Bodies

I like to think of insulin as the mother of all hormones because it impacts and influences all the other endocrine hormones, including the adrenal, sex, and thyroid hormones, all of which we'll go into later.

In school, we were taught that insulin lets blood sugar into the cells so it can be used for energy. When we eat, our body

---

[27] https://smile.amazon.com/Nutrition-Physical-Degeneration-Weston-Price/dp/0916764206/ref=sr_1_1?crid=1P952P4HIS3XC&keywords=nutrition+and+physical+degeneration+by+weston+price&qid=1663775756&sprefix=nutrition+and+%2Caps%2C155&sr=8-1

converts carbohydrates into glucose, which runs around in our bloodstream.[28] Insulin is then released to get glucose into our cells so that they convert to ATP (adenosine triphosphate, or energy).

Your body does not want too much glucose in your blood. Ideally, it wants to keep blood sugar between 70 to 90 mg/dL at all times. While this is a very tight range, the body knows how to keep those numbers in check.

Insulin is the hormone that lowers blood sugar by putting glucose into storage, and it is also a multitasker.[29] When there is extra glucose in the blood, there is a surplus of fuel to use, so insulin sends a message to the rest of the body not to release any because it has enough energy running around in the form of high blood sugar.[30,31] Fat deposits—saddlebags, muffin tops, and so on—are storage fuel and where the excess glucose is stored as fat (or triglycerides, to be exact).

---

[28] https://www.cambridge.org/core/journals/british-journal-of-nutrition/article/associations-between-postprandial-insulin-and-blood-glucose-responses-appetite-sensations-and-energy-intake-in-normal-weight-and-overweight-individuals-a-metaanalysis-of-test-meal-studies/ACB46EA3F14946584DA4F420B2D27705

[29] https://www.nih.gov/news-events/news-releases/nih-study-shows-how-insulin-stimulates-fat-cells-take-glucose

[30] M. D. Jensen, M. Caruso, V. Hailing, and J. M. Miles, "Insulin Regulation of Lipolysis in Nondiabetic and IDDM Subjects," *Diabetes* 38 (1989), 1595–1601.

[31] S. D. Phinney, B. R. Bistrian, R. R. Wolfe, and G. L. Blackburn, "The Human Metabolic Response to Chronic Ketosis without Caloric Restriction: Physical and Biochemical Adaptation," *Metabolism* 32 (1983), 757–768.

This means that if your insulin is raised, it is not possible to lose fat, because your body is being told by insulin not to let any fat out of storage.[32]

Let that resonate with you for a few minutes, because it made me mad when I first heard it. Over the decades, I tried to lose weight, according to standard guidelines. I was told to eat lots of frequent meals with carbohydrates and protein but avoid fat.

> If your insulin is raised, it is not possible to lose fat, because your body is being told by insulin not to let any fat out of storage.

Think about it—if you eat carbs every two to three hours, what is insulin doing to the fat stores that you're trying to lose? It's literally not possible to lose weight if insulin is always being released and telling your body not to allow your fat to get used unless you are just going into a state of starvation.

If you tried to create a diet to gain weight, you couldn't do a better job than the guidelines that they give us. If you're mad like I was, use that frustration to make better choices for the future. Let's get into how to do that.

MANAGING INSULIN SPIKES

What we need is to get and keep our insulin low, which we can accomplish by not eating foods that cause blood sugar to rise,

---

[32] https://smile.amazon.com/Obesity-Code-Unlocking-Secrets-Weight/dp/1771641258/ref=sr_1_2_sspa?crid=DLL24R0Y9QA1&keywords=fung&qid=1663776624&sprefix=fung%2Caps%2C226&sr=8-2-spons&psc=1&spLa=ZW5jcnlwdGVkUXVhbGlmaWVyPUFPWUFBVEo3UVZJVlQmZW5jcnlwdGVkSWQ9QTEwNDI1OTQxSlBQOVFaUjgwVVY4JmVuY3J5cHRlZEFkSWQ9QTA1NzY3MzIySFBYUUNLMDRQQlZJJndpZGdldE5hbWU9c3BfYXRmJmFjdGlvbj1jbGlja1JlZGlyZWN0JmRvTm90TG9nQ2xpY2s9dHJ1ZQ==

which would then trigger insulin to be released. Low carb and ketogenic diets that have finally become popular are spot on.

However, I want you to focus on not just lowering carbs, but the *why* behind it. With your insulin high, you can't burn fat, and that's the key to losing weight.

Diabetics know this is true because they know that they gain weight when they are put on insulin.[33,34,35] Weight gain is inevitable because insulin tells our bodies that they should not release any of our fat stores, and it just adds to those stores.

We have shifted the proportions and the timing of what we eat in recent years according to our crazy government guidelines.[36] We are encouraged to have high glucose because we're constantly getting it in "typical American foods"—it's in the cereal, sandwiches, spaghetti, and pizza that we eat all the time.

Most foods are composed of each of the macronutrients—protein, carbohydrates, and fat. Our bodies are like hybrid cars in that we should ideally shift back and forth between fuel sources (i.e., burning carbohydrates and fat for fuel).[37,38,39]

Because we are told to eat every few hours, we never really get to the point where we can burn fat, so we pretty much lose the ability to do it, and we instinctively want the blood sugar spike, so we eat more carbs. All that fat gets stored as saddlebags, beer bellies, and muffin tops because we have an unlimited storage capacity for it.

---

[33] https://doi.org/10.1016/S1262-3636(05)88268-0
[34] https://journals.sagepub.com/doi/abs/10.1177/0145721706294259
[35] https://doi.org/10.1016/j.diabres.2004.07.005
[36] https://www.myplate.gov/
[37] https://journals.physiology.org/doi/full/10.1152/ajpendo.90558.2008
[38] https://onlinelibrary.wiley.com/doi/abs/10.1111/j.1467-789X.2008.00544.x
[39] https://www.cambridge.org/core/journals/proceedings-of-the-nutrition-society/article/metabolic-flexibility/6649F3D8E24414FD6997DBFEAE8A090E

It may stand to reason that if you just don't eat fat, you'll lose weight, but over the long term, when people do this, they end up eating more carbohydrates. If you only focus on eating carbs, you will always have too much insulin running around putting the glucose away for storage. When you eat fat, it doesn't cause much insulin to be released, especially in comparison to carbohydrates.[40] Additionally, excess blood glucose is converted into molecules called triglycerides when it is stored as fat.[41] So, fat is mainly created by insulin storing carbs as triglycerides.

Another interesting point that I find fascinating is that there are NO essential carbohydrates.[42] "Essential" means that you have to have them to live, and your body can't make them. There are essential amino acids which are the building blocks of proteins, and there are essential fatty acids, like Omega-3s and Omega-6s—your body has to get them from your diet and can't make them. It also can't make minerals and vitamins; you have to purposely take them in. But there are no essential carbohydrates. However, you can make carbohydrates in a process called *gluconeogenesis*, which allows your body to create glucose out of proteins or fats.[43]

> There are NO essential carbohydrates.

Now, why in the world would your body do this? Know that it is so beautifully designed that it doesn't do it for fun, and it doesn't do it by chance. Everything it does is strategic and in your best interest because that is how it was designed.

---

[40] https://academic.oup.com/jcem/article-abstract/66/2/323/2653804
[41] https://www.sciencedirect.com/science/article/abs/pii/S1043276008001379
[42] https://doi.org/10.1093/ajcn/75.5.951a
[43] https://doi.org/10.1016/0026-0495(72)90028-5

The body goes through the gluconeogenesis process because it always wants to keep the blood sugar between 70 and 90 mg/dL.[44] Gluconeogenesis is just one of several mechanisms to ensure this. So, you don't have to eat carbs to keep your blood sugar up—your body can do it on its own.

It is actually more dangerous to have low blood sugar than it is to have high blood sugar. You can see this when you study the hormones and realize that so many raise blood sugar. Glucagon, adrenaline (epinephrine), noradrenaline (norepinephrine), and cortisol all do this directly.[45,46] Additionally, there are even more that raise blood sugar indirectly such as ghrelin, ACTH, thyroid hormones, aldosterone, human growth hormone, and other culprits.

Only one hormone, insulin, will lower the blood sugar.

> Only one hormone, insulin, will lower the blood sugar.

---

[44] https://doi.org/10.1111/nyas.13435
[45] https://www.endocrineweb.com/conditions/diabetes/normal-regulation-blood-glucose
[46] https://en.wikipedia.org/wiki/Blood_sugar_regulation

Hormones That Regulate Blood Sugar

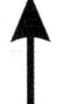

Increase Blood Sugar
- **Glucagon - pancreas**
- Cortisol — adrenals
- Epinephrine — adrenals
- Norepinephrine — adrenals
- Several other minor hormones

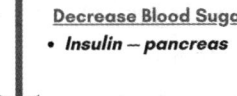

Decrease Blood Sugar
- *Insulin — pancreas*

"Never before in the history of the world have we had an emergency need to LOWER blood sugar, that is until we started to consume large amounts of refined carbohydrates/sugars."
—Gray Graham, founder of Nutritional Therapy Association

Figure 3-1: Hormones to raise/lower blood sugar

Does that seem a little disproportionate to you? It stuck out like a flashing red light to me when I went through my nutritional training.

The body is usually very balanced in how it works. We already talked about how when a joint moves, there are two or three muscles that create motion on either side of the joint, opposing each other. If there's a process that the hormones need to control, there are usually two or three hormones opposing and regulating each other. In other words, there are always backup systems.

The process of regulating blood sugar is dramatically different and should warrant our attention and investigation. The body sees it as drastically more important to keep our blood sugar up, but from where we are standing, it seems to need more mechanisms to get it down. (In the next chapter, you're going see how all chronic disease comes from having high blood sugar.)

If you look into the history of humankind and the food supply, you'll find that it's only been in the last two hundred years or so that we've had access to foods that raise our blood sugar—this is what Weston Price was talking about when he said the "foods of modern civilization" were causing tooth decay and poor health.[47]

Processed Carbohydrates in the Modern Diet

Before the Industrial Revolution, we didn't have much access to white flour, sugar, and other processed foods. These foods were so expensive that they were consumed in vastly lower quantities, and for the most part, no one other than royalty had access to them. This makes sense when you read history books and find that the rich commonly suffered from gout, which is driven by blood sugar imbalances.

Did you know that the average American consumes over 150 pounds of sugar per year?[48] This doesn't take into account other carbohydrates we consume, like white flour.

Would it surprise you to know that eating sugar and processed flour (aka white flour) actually costs your body nutrients in order to digest them?[49] They are anti-nutrients because the body has to supply nutrients from its own stores in order to digest them. This is a net negative effect.

This is not a matter of our bodies being broken—we've simply screwed up our food supply, and in modern society, we have to be intentional to work against this and correct it. It's a daunting task, but it is possible—that's the good news.

---

[47] https://onlinestatbook.com/2/case_studies/sugar.html
[48] https://sugarscience.ucsf.edu/dispelling-myths-too-much.html#.Yys_43bMJD8
[49] https://doi.org/10.1093/ajcn/62.1.203S

At this point, you may wonder why you should eat carbs at all.

There are good reasons to eat certain carbs. Carbs provide fiber, which—while we can't digest it—feeds our good gut bacteria.[50] This fiber comes from plant sources (i.e., vegetables) and is not available anywhere else. Research has shown that diversity in vegetable fiber is the key to having a healthy gut.[51,52,53] You don't want to just eat one form of fiber—you want to have a diversification of fibers to feed the different strains of good bacteria. (There will be more about this in the digestive section of this book.)[54,55,56]

Another reason to eat carbohydrates is for the phytonutrients, which are nutrients that are uniquely found in plant matter and have healing properties.[57] These include curcumin, resveratrol, lutein, flavonoids, zeaxanthin, carotenoids, indoles, ECGC, and many more. You may recognize these nutrients as they are often referred to as *superfoods* and have been shown to have health benefits for addressing cancer and other diseases.[58,59]

What you want to stay away from to keep a low insulin diet are starchy carbs and sugar, not vegetables. While I encourage consumption of an abundance of healthy, low carb vegetables, this is not a vegetarian or vegan approach. This low insulin diet

---

[50] https://doi.org/10.3390/nu5041417
[51] https://doi.org/10.1007/s00394-002-1102-7
[52] https://www.mdpi.com/2073-4425/10/7/534
[53] https://www.ncbi.nlm.nih.gov/pmc/articles/PMC5390821/
[54] https://doi.org/10.1080%2F19490976.2017.1290756
[55] https://doi.org/10.3390%2Fnu13051655
[56] https://doi.org/10.3390%2Fnu12030859
[57] https://link.springer.com/referenceworkentry/10.1007/978-981-13-1745-3_2-1
[58] https://doi.org/10.1016/j.abb.2015.02.018
[59] https://www.mdpi.com/2218-273X/11/8/1176

goes against the plant-based political movement and everything that we've grown up hearing in terms of government guidelines, which can make it really confusing. (If you'd like to dive into this and hear more about the research, history, and politics behind these recommendations, check out Nina Teicholz's book, *The Big Fat Surprise*.)[60]

While it is possible to do a low insulin vegetarian diet, it is extremely difficult, and a low insulin vegan diet is impossible because you would be restricted to only plants for protein, which will have a lot of carbs and bring on the insulin. Additionally, a vegan or vegetarian diet is going to leave you deficient in nutrients because they are not as bioavailable to your body as animal nutrient forms.[61]

For example, carrots may be high in beta carotene, but it is not actually vitamin A (retinol)—it's a carotenoid which is a precursor to vitamin A that your body has to make into vitamin A, and up to 45 percent of females can't make this conversion.[62,63,64] While someone may think they are getting plenty of vitamin A with all the carrots they eat, they may not be able to convert it and are left in a vitamin A-deficient state. Eating clean meat will give you a bioavailable form of vitamin A from an animal that already did the conversion process for you.[65] (Gotta love those thoughtful cows!)

---

[60] https://smile.amazon.com/Big-Fat-Surprise-Butter-Healthy-ebook/dp/B00A25FDUA/ref=sr_1_3?crid=2O8T6TPM2C7JN&keywords=nina+teicholz&qid=1663781665&s=books&sprefix=nina+tie%2Cstripbooks%2C231&sr=1-3

[61] https://smile.amazon.com/Vegetarianism-Explained-Making-Informed-Decision/dp/0954852060/ref=sr_1_1?crid=1RIW5DIJABQ03&keywords=vegetarian+natasha+campbell+mcbride&qid=1663781709&s=books&sprefix=vegetarian+natasha+campbell+mcbride%2Cstripbooks%2C155&sr=1-1

[62] https://onlinelibrary.wiley.com/doi/full/10.1002/jsfa.2647

[63] https://doi.org/10.3945/jn.111.140756

[64] https://faseb.onlinelibrary.wiley.com/doi/abs/10.1096/fj.08-121962

[65] https://www.ncbi.nlm.nih.gov/pmc/articles/PMC4785134/

Eating a low insulin diet is not a new fad—it actually brings us back to how our bodies were designed to eat and how all our ancestors ate until the Industrial Revolution. A low insulin diet will help you keep your eye on the goal of getting your hormones balanced, and lowering your carbohydrate intake is what will get you there.

The ketogenic diet—which falls into this category—has been around for over a hundred years and has been used for therapeutic purposes for everything from epilepsy (which is what it was originally designed for) to diabetes to cancer.[66] It hasn't gotten the attention that it should have received until recently because, quite frankly, it cuts out the need for pharmaceuticals.

There are no long-term ill effects in using a low carb or ketogenic diet, and people have been eating this way for decades.[67] Yes, there are some areas where you'll want to be strategic as you shift into a state where your insulin is lowered, and we'll problem-solve that in the following chapters.

Insulin is hard on the body. Not only can you not release fat stores, but when you have high insulin, it means that there's a lot of glucose running around your body. When glucose is high in your blood, it coats your proteins and creates what are called *advanced glycation end products* (AGEs). These AGEs are a huge driver of inflammation in your body, which is going to affect your joints and set all the big chronic diseases in motion.[68]

---

[66] https://doi.org/10.1111/j.1528-1167.2008.01821.x
[67] https://doi.org/10.7759%2Fcureus.9639
[68] https://doi.org/10.4093/dmj.2017.0105

Chapter 4
Heading Off Chronic Disease at the Pass

I don't look like a typical Pilates instructor. All my life, I've struggled with carrying that extra 20 pounds, and no matter how much Pilates I did, it was always there. The worst part was that I could see the look in a potential client's eyes as they asked themselves, *Why in the world would I take lessons from her when she's overweight?*

I always wanted to explain that I was a great teacher because Pilates is about joint health, not weight, but since weight loss was often inappropriately their goal, the idea fell flat. This broke my heart, but what I didn't know then is what I am desperate to share with you now.

EXTRA WEIGHT AND A BIGGER PROBLEM

In current society, no one connects how today's symptoms lead to tomorrow's disease. They look at them as separate issues in and of themselves. Our standard of care won't diagnose an issue until it becomes a disease state, when it could have been prevented if it had been addressed earlier.[69] They aren't even looking for the root cause of the symptoms that we come into their offices complaining about.

For example, if you tell a doctor that you want to lose weight, what are they going to tell you? They won't talk about insulin, but they'll tell you how you need to lower your calories and eat less fat, even though this has been disproven.[70]

The bigger problem is the diseases for which the doctors have no cure—type 2 diabetes, heart disease, cancer, and Alzheimer's. Symptoms like joint pain and weight gain are things that motivate people to make changes, but they are really early-onset symptoms of bigger, chronic diseases. They need to be identified as such so that we will see that we have power to avoid them.

THE CHRONIC DISEASE SPECTRUM

Disease is not a switch that goes on or off; it's more a slow progression toward dysfunction and complication. The earlier you start to untangle the ball of yarn, the easier it is, and the more likely you will be successful. The first step is to acknowledge and understand that there is a tangle in your yarn up ahead.

---

[69] https://doi.org/10.4093/dmj.2017.0105
[70] Ludwig, David S., and Cara B. Ebbeling. "The carbohydrate-insulin model of obesity: beyond 'calories in, calories out'." *JAMA internal medicine* 178, no. 8 (2018): 1098–1103.

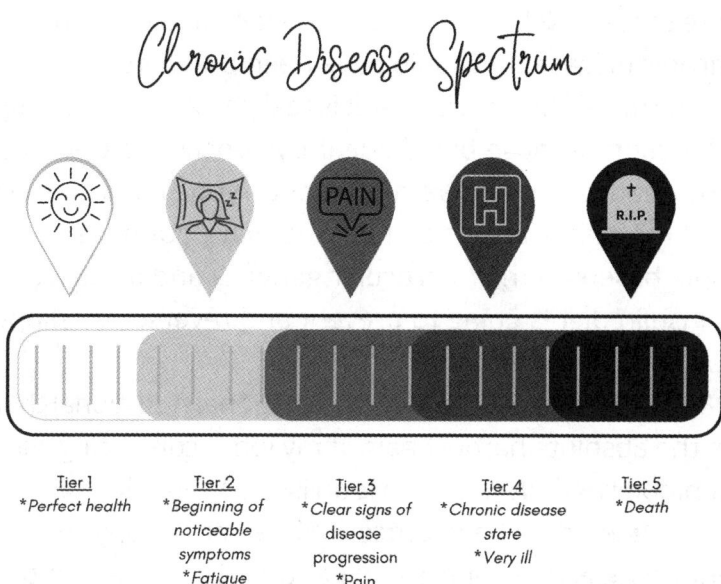

Figure 4-1: Chronic disease spectrum

This means that things like weight gain are your body's way of telling you that something's wrong before there's a diagnosable disease state. If you take heed of these early symptoms, you can save yourself a world of hurt later and prevent your worst fears from coming true.

Now, this isn't the sexy part—no one wants to take preventative measures when you may not even have symptoms. Who wants to pay for tests, organic food, supplements, and more if they aren't necessary? You won't know if they are necessary until you run tests, or you can just wait until it is too late, and you have Alzheimer's or cancer.

When using the QR code at the end of the Introduction, you will find a free tool so that you can begin to understand where you are on the chronic disease spectrum. This will give you motivation to do something now and a clear direction of where to start. Now is the time to take action before you have a chronic disease that could have been prevented.

In terms of chronic disease, it is really all about blood sugar dysfunction because blood sugar dysfunction is the root of all the deadly chronic diseases that everyone fears—yes, you heard me right—and this one issue plays out differently in people based on their particular genetics and lifestyle.[71,72] A low insulin diet is going to prevent and reverse the slippery slope into chronic disease.

But here's the problem—as a functional nutritional therapist, the absolute hardest part of my job is convincing clients that blood sugar dysfunction is an issue. When do they come to me? When they have cancer. While I am happy to help a client address their illness and get their body back on track, wouldn't it be lovely if they had come in several years to a decade before and prevented the whole issue altogether? That's where my passion is, and that's where I want to empower you to take control of your life and do the preventative work so you don't have to figure this out the way I did.

Now, if you think that this isn't you and you don't have a problem, I get it. This is the area people will fight me on; then we get the labs back and look at their food journals and, lo and behold, they see it. I can't emphasize enough that you don't feel bad when your blood sugar is high.

> You don't feel bad when your blood sugar is high.

---

[71] https://diabetesjournals.org/diabetes/article/37/12/1595/8592/Role-of-Insulin-Resistance-in-Human-Disease

[72] https://smile.amazon.com/Real-Food-Keto-Jimmy-Moore-ebook/dp/B09PLKRSPY/ref=sr_1_1?crid=FEVGCOFOGRPX&keywords=real+food+keto&qid=1663785577&s=books&sprefix=real+food+keto%2Cstripbooks%2C178&sr=1-1

To the mamas out there—you have a very special role, and you can be the hero in your family. Moms can not only prevent their own chronic disease, but they also hold the reins for their entire family. Who does the grocery shopping, the meal planning, the lunch packing, and the outing planning? Those things are all going to be what feeds and drives the blood sugar dysregulation or corrects it in all the members of your family. If you choose well for them and educate them on the how and why behind their food choices, you have set them up for life—and the lives of generations beyond them.

This may make you cringe, but I think it is important to say. We, as a culture and as individuals, need to start calling out truth. Letting your child know that you aren't going to be giving them candy because it is a poison (and you love them more than that) is huge.[73] Yes, poison—does that make you cringe? We need to shift our worldview and that of our children and how they view food. We need to understand that food can be a tool for good or harm.

I just really want to point out that you've got more power than you think. If you have older kids who are more set in their ways and are being influenced by peers, you can blame your changes on me—I would be honored to be thrown under the bus in the name of health!

Chronic Diseases to Avoid

Let's dive into what chronic health conditions you'll want to sidestep, so that you are well armed when you feel resistant to change or are offered a gooey cupcake.

---

[73] https://www.ncbi.nlm.nih.gov/pmc/articles/PMC6959843/

Type 2 diabetes—Mary came to me because she thought she had some odd symptoms and wanted to feel less tired. She needed to pee often, seemed thirsty all the time, and sometimes had numbness in her feet. She was scared that she might have diabetes, and it sounded likely when we discussed what she regularly ate—lots of healthy whole grains. We did an at-home version of an oral glucose tolerance test, and it pointed strongly toward her suspicions.

Type 2 diabetes is completely reversible with diet, but Mary didn't really believe it because she had never heard that before.[74] She was willing to try to change things, so we discussed what a low insulin diet looked like and problem-solved some areas.

Mary was on a very tight budget and concerned that it would cost too much, but I explained that while you'll eat more expensive ingredients, you'll be eating less of them, so the cost doesn't need to be more if you economize. (I have lots of tricks for this—remember, I have seven kids!) We started with diet alone, nothing else. She was not strict with it because—let's face it—carbs are cheap, and that's what she had been used to eating.

She gradually got off carbs and reversed the situation within a matter of months. The best part was that her "weird" symptoms all went away, and her energy came back. She had even lost that extra 10 pounds that she had been struggling with for years. She was ecstatic, although she didn't fully understand the pothole that she had sidestepped in terms of diabetes complications—foot amputations, glaucoma, kidney

---

[74] https://www.ncbi.nlm.nih.gov/pmc/articles/PMC6520897/

disease, oral health issues, hearing loss, heart disease, obesity, and the like.[75]

Do you know what the treatment for diabetes is with our current standard of care? They give you insulin, even though it drives all those awful side effects and makes the problem worse. When you eat carbs, you're given insulin so they will get put into storage, and your blood sugar lowers. Having more insulin is why type 2 diabetics gain weight.[76]

After what I explained in the last chapter, I think you can clearly see that giving someone more insulin, while it will help in the short term (immediately after a meal), is very hard on the body in the long term. The bottom line is that they don't think you are smart enough or self-disciplined enough to fix the problem through diet, but I know you are! If you get the insulin lowered, there won't be a need for extra insulin because there isn't high blood glucose to get down.

This is also true for type 1 diabetics as well, although they will still need some insulin and need to monitor their blood sugar closely.[77] They can drastically reduce their need for it (and the cost) with a low insulin diet. Not only does this make things cheaper in terms of buying insulin, but it also prevents advanced glycation end products from running rampant due to their blood sugar being high all the time and causing lots of damage. Doctors never tell them this, however, which I don't understand.[78]

---

[75] https://www.mayoclinic.org/diseases-conditions/type-2-diabetes/symptoms-causes/syc-20351193
[76] https://www.mayoclinic.org/diseases-conditions/type-2-diabetes/symptoms-causes/syc-20351193
[77] https://www.ccjm.org/content/88/10/547
[78] https://www.cdc.gov/diabetes/managing/eat-well/meal-plan-method.html

Heart disease—Heidi came to me with serious concerns about her high cholesterol numbers. She was thinking that she was following in the path of her father, who had died of a heart attack.

When I took a look at her labs, her lipid panel was off the charts. She had high cholesterol and all the different facets of it. However, that is not what I was concerned about with her when I talked to her about her eating. It was clear that she had a very high carb diet, and when I explained to her how this was connected to her cholesterol markers, she was shocked because her doctor had not mentioned this to her. He just wanted to put her on statins. I also went a step further and told her that we should run some thyroid tests—if you have a sluggish thyroid, it often contributes to high cholesterol numbers.[79]

Well, we ran the thyroid tests, and it turned out she was hypothyroid (she had a sluggish thyroid). We worked on a low insulin diet for her along with some thyroid support. Not only did she lose 25 pounds, but she also felt better, and her cholesterol numbers came down very nicely and easily without doing anything specifically for her cholesterol. We simply addressed the root issues.

I told Heidi that every time she ate carbs and her blood sugar went up, there were advanced glycation end products that were being formed in her body. As I mentioned earlier, AGEs arise when sugars glycate onto proteins and lipids in your blood—they damage them. At this point, proteins/fats become a kind of hard molecule that loses its flexibility. As it runs around in the blood, it's nicking the sides of the blood vessels and causing damage to those too. The body knows

---

[79] Duntas, Leonidas H., and Leonard Wartofsky. "Cardiovascular risk and subclinical hypothyroidism: focus on lipids and new emerging risk factors. What is the evidence?" *Thyroid* 17, no. 11 (2007): 1075–1084.

this is not good, so it will send the repair team out, which is cholesterol.[80]

The cholesterol goes to work to make a patch over the injured site so it can be repaired.[81] Think of it like temporary walls around areas of construction along a busy street. Cholesterol really isn't the bad guy here—it's the good guy![82] It's like someone observing that firefighters are always at house fires but jumping to the conclusion that they are causing the house fire. It's not the firefighter (i.e., the cholesterol) causing the damage—they are there to help repair it.

Here's the interesting part—so we hear that we need to avoid eating cholesterol, but did you know that your body makes up to 60 percent of your cholesterol? Giving a statin drug to stop you from making your own cholesterol is handicapping your body from making its own repair team and worsening the situation.[83,84] What you want to do is get to the root issue and address the blood sugar that is causing those damaging glycation end products to run rampant throughout your system in the first place.

---

[80] Campbell-McBride, Natasha. *Put Your Heart in Your Mouth: Natural Treatment for Atherosclerosis, Angina, Heart Attack, High Blood Pressure, Stroke, Arrhythmia, Peripheral Vascular Disease*. Medinform Publishing; 1st edition (March 2, 2016)

[81] https://smile.amazon.com/Cholesterol-Clarity-Jimmy-Moore-ebook/dp/B09PLL7SHS/ref=sr_1_1?crid=12WT4PLRBRKYG&keywords=what+the+hdl&qid=1663787182&s=books&sprefix=what+the+hdl%2Cstripbooks%2C223&sr=1-1

[82] Campbell-McBride, Natasha. *Put Your Heart in Your Mouth: Natural Treatment for Atherosclerosis, Angina, Heart Attack, High Blood Pressure, Stroke, Arrhythmia, Peripheral Vascular Disease*. Medinform Publishing; 1st edition (March 2, 2016)

[83] Yebyo, H. G., Aschmann, H. E., Puhan, M. A. "Finding the balance between benefits and harms when using statins for primary prevention of cardiovascular disease." [published online December 4, 2018]. *Ann Intern Med*. 2018; DOI: 10.7326/M18-1279.

[84] Richman, I. B., Ross, J. S. "Weighing the harms and benefits of using statins for primary prevention: raising the risk threshold." [published online December 4, 2018]. *Ann Intern Med*. 2018; DOI: 10.7326/M18-3066.

By the way, there are better markers than looking at a lipid panel—it is just the cheap test that insurance typically wants to run. But looking at your apolipoprotein ratios and your hs-CRP is going to give you a much better idea of where you're at, and as I mentioned before, I would also run some blood sugar tests and full thyroid panel to see how those are contributing to the situation.[85,86,87]

Cancer—I already mentioned that I had a journey with breast cancer, but I want to tell you a little bit about the context of the situation.

When I found out that I had breast cancer, I was postpartum with my fifth child. This was after I had already learned a little bit about diet and thought I was taking care of my body (but I wasn't a nutritionist yet). Our family had been doing some intense gut work with a diet called *gut and psychology syndrome* (GAPS).

With the GAPS diet, all grains and a lot of carbohydrates were eliminated.[88] However, I did not know that I had blood sugar dysfunction at that time—I was perfectly able to maintain my insulin resistance and blood sugar dysregulation with healthy foods like honey, beans, squash, and fruit. Insulin resistance is when the cells of the body don't want any more glucose, but the body keeps making more insulin to try and force it in.[89] It was on the spectrum toward diabetes, but I felt completely fine.

Now that I understand blood sugar, I can look back and see these patterns, but I couldn't see them at the time because I

---

[85] https://pubmed.ncbi.nlm.nih.gov/14746556/
[86] https://www.ncbi.nlm.nih.gov/pmc/articles/PMC8540246/
[87] https://www.ncbi.nlm.nih.gov/pmc/articles/PMC4825196/
[88] Campbell-McBride, Natasha. *Gut and Psychology Syndrome: Natural Treatment for Autism, Dyspraxia, A.D.D., Dyslexia, A.D.H.D., Depression, Schizophrenia.* Medinform Publishing; Revised & enlarged edition (November 15, 2010)
[89] https://www.ncbi.nlm.nih.gov/pmc/articles/PMC1204764/

didn't know what I know now. I had no idea that I was setting myself up for cancer.

What I hear all the time from my cancer clients is, "I never saw this coming." Well, here's the real deal—no one ever sees cancer coming because it doesn't feel bad to have blood sugar dysregulation, and no one is talking about the fact that cancer is a metabolic disease.

The defining sign of determining cancer is when a cell has shifted metabolically. This occurs when the cell's mitochondria (where energy is produced in the cell) switches from aerobic to anaerobic.[90] This is called the *Warburg effect*—it was discovered back in 1931, so it is not a new concept at all. When this happens, the mitochondria stop using the citric acid cycle (aka the Krebs cycle) to burn fuel sources and anaerobically use only glucose, not oxygen.[91] This is a very inefficient way to function, and that shift means that the cell needs two hundred times as much glucose as a normal cell to be able to function.[92]

Therefore, by addressing the metabolic dysfunction of the cancer cells' mitochondria and not feeding it the high levels of glucose it desperately wants, you are able to shift things back and put the cancer in remission.[93,94]

This is the major reason, but there are always additional contributing factors that create the terrain for cancer to

---

[90] en.wikipedia.org/wiki/Warburg_effect_(oncology)
[91] Seyfried, Thomas. *Cancer as a Metabolic Disease: On the Origin, Management, and Prevention of Cancer 1st Edition.* Wiley; 1st edition (June 26, 2012).
[92] Rath, Linda. "Cancer and Sugar: Is There a Link?" Medically Reviewed by Melinda Ratini, DO, MS on February 12, 2019
[93] Winters, Dr. Nasha, ND FABNO L.Ac Dipl.OM, and Kelley, Jess Higgins, MNT. Turner, Kelly (Foreword). *The Metabolic Approach to Cancer: Integrating Deep Nutrition, the Ketogenic Diet, and Nontoxic Bio-Individualized Therapies.* Chelsea Green Publishing (May 24, 2017)
[94] Seyfried, Thomas. *Cancer as a Metabolic Disease: On the Origin, Management, and Prevention of Cancer* 1st Edition. Wiley; 1st edition (June 26, 2012)

thrive—it is never just one thing, and all of it needs to be addressed.[95]

I want to highlight that cancer is a metabolic disease that needs to be addressed to get to the root of why the body was not able to address the cancer itself the way that it is designed to. If you address the blood sugar dysregulation before you get cancer, you're sidestepping a huge pothole.[96] The low insulin/ketogenic diet is the absolute first thing I do with my cancer clients. There will be individual tweaks, but overall, they must address the metabolic dysfunction.

Another aspect that you want to think about with cancer is that if you are overweight, your fat is actually considered its own endocrine organ.[97] That means that your fat is actually producing hormones on its own.[98,99] So, your saddlebags, beer belly, muffin top, and so on are actually producing estrogens. Most people are familiar with the idea that a lot of cancers are driven by hormones that are out of control—it's one of those other contributing factors I alluded to.

This needs to be discussed in our age of body positivity. Hear me out before you get mad at me. While I do believe that everyone is beautifully made in the image of God, I don't believe that being fat is beautiful. It's unhealthy and a sign

---

[95] Winters, Dr. Nasha, ND FABNO L.Ac Dipl.OM, and Kelley, Jess Higgins, MNT. Turner, Kelly (Foreword). *The Metabolic Approach to Cancer: Integrating Deep Nutrition, the Ketogenic Diet, and Nontoxic Bio-Individualized Therapies*. Chelsea Green Publishing (May 24, 2017)

[96] https://smile.amazon.com/Fat-Fuel-Revolutionary-Combat-Increase-ebook/dp/B06W2KVK1P/ref=sr_1_1?crid=2NEXG626XZ8NE&keywords=fat+for+fuel&qid=1663796774&s=books&sprefix=fat+for+fuel%2Cstripbooks%2C388&sr=1-1

[97] https://doi.org/10.1016/0960-0760(94)90274-7

[98] https://www.sciencedirect.com/science/article/abs/pii/S0303720717304999

[99] https://doi.org/10.1210/edrv-10-2-136

that you need to make changes. I love the person, and I want them to be healthy.

It's the same as if someone had all their hair fall out because their thyroid was messed up or if someone's skin turned bright red and peeled from a sunburn —these are things that indicate that you need to make some different choices, such as supporting your thyroid or limiting sun exposure. It doesn't mean we should judge, criticize, or think less of these people. We need to love them and help them optimize their body's function.

Dementia—As I write this, I'm staying in Phoenix visiting my dad, who is in a memory care facility, while my mom is out of town. He has type 3 diabetes, which is more commonly known as Alzheimer's (or its generic name, dementia). He had a stroke a couple of months ago. It left him unable to walk, and my mom could no longer take care of him on her own.

It's heartbreaking to see a once vibrant, strong man be humbled in this drastic way to where he can't even remember what I told him yesterday, or what I told him five minutes ago, for that matter. It kills me to watch my dad struggle with this when I know it is preventable, but I didn't know this when it should have been addressed. I cry the whole way home every day, and I'm begging you to take heed so that no one you love ends up like my dad.

Research has shown that dementia is a metabolic dysfunction—mitochondria are not working properly, and blood sugar is rampantly dysregulated.[100,101] It's hard to see because you

---

[100] https://doi.org/10.1177/193229680800200619
[101] https://doi.org/10.1016/j.bbadis.2016.08.018

don't feel bad having high insulin levels, but it takes its toll on your body, especially your brain.

Prevention is the only way to confront dementia. Once you have it, you may be able to slow it down, so start yesterday! When you have some of those early memory issues, don't dismiss them as just getting old—this is not normal. Look at your blood sugar and address your diet and lifestyle.[102] The time to prevent Alzheimer's is decades before it starts—this is the message I want to get out. Yes, you can slow things down. But the only cure is to prevent it.

All of these major killers are preventable. The monster in the closet has just been exposed, and if you take away its insulin, it will melt into thin air. The common factor in each is blood sugar dysregulation, and it is not what anyone, even your doctor, is talking about.[103]

Furthermore, no one wants to hear about it because, deep down, we don't think it will happen to us since we don't feel bad. So, we stick our heads in the sand and say, "I'll think about that tomorrow."

But trust me—tomorrow comes fast when you're not looking.

---

[102] https://smile.amazon.com/Reversing-Alzheimers-Prevent-Dementia-Revitalize/dp/173504802X/ref=sr_1_1?crid=2TLWEEDQBMRBI&keywords=timothy+smith+alzheimer%27s&qid=1663797180&s=books&sprefix=timothy+smith+alzheimer%27s%2Cstripbooks%2C172&sr=1-1

[103] https://smile.amazon.com/End-Alzheimers-Program-Prevent-Cognitive-ebook/dp/B01M28ROCU/ref=sr_1_1?crid=H6VZ0RZXTLR5&keywords=end+of+alzheimer%27s+by+dale+bredesen&qid=1663797207&s=books&sprefix=alzheimer%27s+bredes%2Cstripbooks%2C172&sr=1-1

Chapter 5
The Importance of Diet

When Jamie came to me, she was unique in that she already understood that she needed to address her blood sugar. However, her reaction was very common. She threw an adult version of a tantrum because she did not want to give up carbs—period. For her, bread was the ultimate thing, and she could not imagine life without it.

She enjoyed cookies and other fun treats regularly, and the idea of not having those was horrifying to her. She literally said that her life would not be worth living without them, which I thought was a little dramatic. I explained to her that she could still have fun treats and keep her insulin down without feeling deprived.[104]

She didn't buy it, but she knew that there was enough of an issue so she agreed to try another way for three months. I gave her resources, recipes, and ideas, and she started her journey reluctantly.

---

[104] https://smile.amazon.com/Ultimate-Guide-Keto-Baking/dp/1628603844/ref=sr_1_5?crid=358EJJ37KV9BP&keywords=carolyn+ketchum+keto+cookbook&qid=1663797285&s=books&sprefix=carolyn+ketc%2Cstripbooks%2C170&sr=1-5

Our Ongoing Love Affair with Carbs

Most people are so used to depending on carbs as the base of their meals that they can't imagine life without them. Think about it—all the restaurants, cooking shows, fun events, holidays—nearly every part of the American diet is based around carbs.

To pull away from carbs seems horrifying, overwhelming, and just not possible. When people make this transition, they feel like they're going to miss out on so many aspects of life and just be tortured. They are used to having carbs fill the gap, not only in awkward social situations but also when they have energy and mood dips.

What they don't realize is that, without carbs, they won't have energy issues in the first place.

The other concern that many people have is that it's going to be way too expensive to upend their diets—especially moms, who must think about transitioning with the whole family. If they can't convert the whole family, they'll have two different diets going on, which is just pure overwhelm and anxiety.

Mamas, please know that your kids will thrive on a low insulin diet. Just make sure they get enough fat because if they are hungry between meals, that means they didn't get enough fat at their last meal.

Kids don't need non-essential carbs any more than an adult does. If you are concerned that a family member may be losing weight that they don't have to lose on this diet, make sure they get enough fat. I have worked with a variety of people who just can't keep weight on (athletes, cachexic cancer clients, growing

> Make sure they get enough fat.

children, people with hyperthyroid conditions, and so on), and they all do great on this diet as long as they get enough fat. (Did I say that enough times?) It's hard work to reprogram what we have been indoctrinated with by the government, education, advertising, and the media.

When you're following a low insulin lifestyle, you are satiated more quickly on less volume.[105] You're not eating the same quantities of food that you were, and it doesn't cost as much as you think it would.

My client Anna is very frugal and had this very concern but tried a low insulin diet, as she was desperate to lose postpartum weight. When she started making fathead (high fat/low carb) pizza for her family, she was shocked that they ate about half the amount they did when she made pizza before. When she did the math, it came out to be about the same price for the healthier, low insulin version, and her family loved it. Win-win!

When trying a low insulin diet, give it a solid three months to see how you feel on the other side. Now, this means that you'll want to really dive in and make it your own—don't just grab little things here and there so that you never actually like it and you don't want to continue.

When I started this lifestyle, there were very few available products out there to support it. For example, basic ingredients for cooking, like almond flour and sweeteners, were not sold at places like Costco and Walmart. Now, I get so excited every time I go to the store because there are keto versions of all of my favorites, including ice cream, chips, cookies, and chocolate! So, do not stress about losing your favorite food items. You can find healthier versions of your favorites!

---

[105] https://www.ncbi.nlm.nih.gov/books/NBK53550/

PUTTING A LOW CARB PLAN INTO ACTION

The basic idea around taking the carbs out is replacing them with fats. Now, I want to encourage you not to take low carb vegetables out because these are going to give you phytonutrients and fiber. I explain to my clients that the low carb (non-starchy) veggies are the base on which to put the fats because no one wants to eat a spoonful of mayonnaise.

Especially at the beginning, getting more fats in your diet will need to be conscious and intentional. If you don't get enough fat, you won't get the fuel your body needs, and this plan will not be sustainable—you'll be constantly hungry, and no one wants that!

Unless you are massively overweight, getting enough fat is imperative. If you are very overweight, getting enough fat won't be as important as you lose weight. The longest known fast was by Angus Barbieri—he went 382 days without eating and went from 456 pounds to 180 pounds.[106] He didn't die without carbs—instead, his body lived off of his own stored fuel source, his fat. However, that's probably not you, so you'll need to supply your body with some fat to burn as fuel. While keeping your insulin levels low, your body will burn your own fat for its fuel source along with your food. It's exciting to have control over this, isn't it?

Did you know that the human body is made up primarily of water, fat, protein, and minerals? There is very little carbohydrate that is stored in our bodies. Besides being a storage pantry for fuel, fats have many vital jobs, such as being made into hormones, prostaglandins, cell membranes, brain and

---

[106] Keenan, Stephen, BFoodSc&Nutr, MDietetics. "Comparing the effects of 5:2 intermittent fasting and continuous energy restriction when combined with resistance training on body composition, muscular strength, cardio-metabolic health markers and dietary compliance." (2020).

nerve sheaths, and the like—your brain is literally 60 percent fat.[107]

Fat also makes up the *prostaglandins*, which are mechanisms to control inflammation in your body.[108] Steroid hormones are literally made of cholesterol, and are the building blocks for all the sex hormones. That means they are critical for things like reproduction, appropriate stress hormones, and sex hormone balance (read that as lack of period or menopause symptoms).[109]

Also, every single cell in our bodies is surrounded by a membrane that is made up of a double layer of fats.[110,111] If you don't have enough good fats coming in, these structures will not function properly at a cellular level.

GOOD FATS VS. BAD FATS

We want to make sure that the fats you take in are high quality so that your body runs correctly.[112] Good fats are not dangerous—they're therapeutic and essential, while bad fats are rancid and create more inflammation and disease.

---

[107] Cockburn, F. "Neonatal brain and dietary lipids." *Archives of Disease in Childhood Fetal and Neonatal edition* 70, no. 1 (1994): F1.
[108] https://doi.org/10.2310/jim.0b013e31819aaa76
[109] https://www.ncbi.nlm.nih.gov/pmc/articles/PMC3636985/
[110] https://www.ncbi.nlm.nih.gov/books/NBK26871/
[111] https://www.nih.gov/news-events/nih-research-matters/dietary-fats-influence-endoplasmic-reticulum-membrane
[112] https://www.ncbi.nlm.nih.gov/pmc/articles/PMC7037798/#:~:text=%CF%89%2D3%20fatty%20acids%20(FAs,of%20the%20fatty%20acid%2C%20respectively.

Fat Molecule Structure

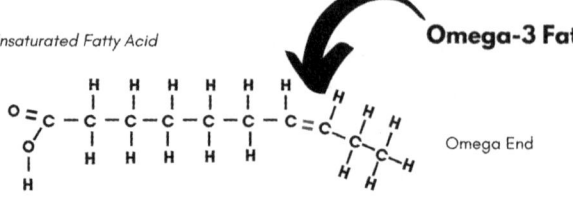

Figure 5-1: Fat molecule

Fat Types and Properties

Fatty Acid	Solid vs Liquid	Rancidity	Cook with?	Examples
Saturated Fat	Fatty acid chain has a single bond and is straight	Solid at room temperature	Hard to go rancid	Very good to cook with	Good Fats: butter, lard, tallow, coconut oil, cocoa butter, full fat heavy cream, full fat cheese, avocados Bad Fats: margarine
Monounsaturated Fat	Fatty acid chain has one double bond and has a slight bend	Liquid at room temperature, but will solidify when cold	Can turn rancid when heated	Should not be heated above 180 degrees	Good Fats: olive oil, avocado oil, sesame oil Bad Fats: canola oil, peanut oil, safflower oil
Polyunsaturated Fat	Fatty acid chain has more than one double bond and is more bent	Liquid at room temperature and is very unstable	Can turn rancid when exposed to light, heat, or air	Never to be cooked with and must be cold-pressed and stored in dark containers	Good Fats: salmon, flaxseed oil Bad Fats: sunflower oil, corn oil, canola oil, soybean oil

Figure 5-2: Properties of different types of fats

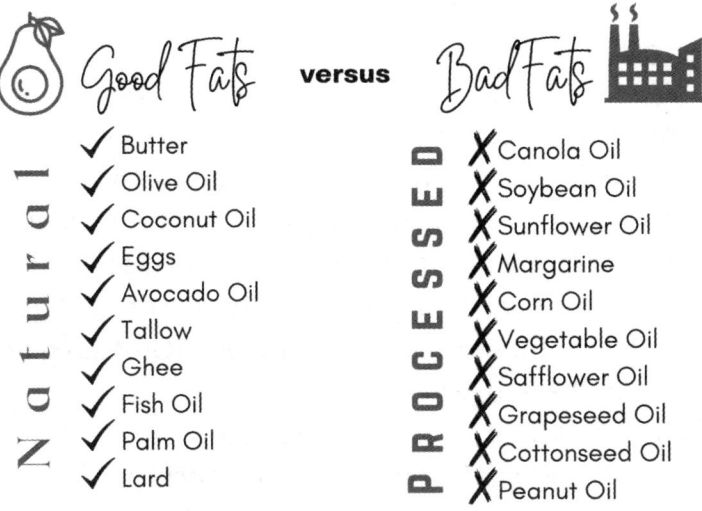

Figure 5-3 : Good fats vs. bad fats

So how do you determine which is which? All fats are made up of a *carboxyl group* (COOH) on one end and a chain of carbons with hydrogens on the other. Whether a fat is good or bad is determined by how the hydrogens are attached to the carbon molecules, and this also affects the properties of the fat and how you want to use it.

We have what we call *saturated*, *monounsaturated*, and *polyunsaturated* fats. Check out the diagram, and you'll see that the saturated fats have all of the spaces filled and are nice and straight. This also means that they pack in tightly together so that they are solid at room temperature and are hard to get to go rancid (i.e., they're great for cooking.)

Monounsaturated fats have only one double bond and have a slight bend to them. They are liquid at room temperature but will solidify when in the fridge. (Since olive oil is a monounsaturated fat and vegetable oils are polyunsaturated, this is a great way to check if your olive oil has been cut with veggie oils.)

Polyunsaturated fats have multiple double bonds and are more bent; they are very unstable and liquid at room temperature. These are fats you never want to cook with.

In the polyunsaturated category are the essential fatty acids (EFAs) that your body can't make, such as Omega-3s and Omega-6s. The name comes from having the first double bond at either three bonds from the end (Omega-3) or six bonds from the end (Omega-6).

Polyunsaturated fats are very delicate, and you only want to consume them if they haven't gone rancid, which occurs when they are exposed to light, heat, or air. If they're in a clear plastic bottle or they've been processed with heat or exposed to air, they are going to be toxic and rancid and are going to do more harm than good by causing inflammation. Run away from these fats—do not let them into your kitchen, do not let them into your mouth, and do not put them on your skin.[113]

The polyunsaturated fat problem started in the early 1900s when we made a massive shift from eating solid animal fats, which were stable and beneficial, to eating polyunsaturated fats, which were created from the waste products of various industries and recycled to give us rancid liquid oils.[114] (They are deodorized and bleached so they don't smell or taste rancid, but trust me, they are.)

The powers that be also discovered how to hydrogenate these fats (i.e., squash some hydrogen on them so they would

---

[113] https://doi.org/10.1146%2Fannurev-nutr-071714-034449
[114] https://smile.amazon.com/Know-Your-Fats-Understanding-Cholesterol/dp/0967812607/ref=sr_1_1?crid=2GNJAUXRTRCLC&keywords=mary+enig&qid=1663800245&s=books&sprefix=mary+enig%2Cstripbooks%2C216&sr=1-1

be straighter, like saturated fats) to create solid rancid fats, like Crisco. We were sold a bill of goods that these fats were good for our hearts and better for us overall, but research has shown the opposite.[115]

Why am I so harsh on polyunsaturated fats? Well, if you really dig into it, you'll find that canola oil and other vegetable oils are all heavily processed, bleached, deodorized, heated, oxidized, and made rancid. These oils need to be protected and babied throughout their processing and transport, but they are not.[116]

I'm not saying the specific oils are bad in and of themselves. If you can find a canola oil that is not genetically modified but that is organically raised without toxins, cold-processed, and kept in a dark glass bottle in the refrigerator, please let me know. (It doesn't exist anywhere—and I've looked!) Make sure that your Omega-3s and -6s are always treated like the gold that they are—cold-pressed and in dark containers—because you want to make sure that the light, heat, and oxygen are not rendering them rancid and undoing all your hard work.

I mentioned "organic" because it is going to be a very important aspect here. I understand that you likely have a budget and that the cost of food is skyrocketing, but when you're eating fat, especially animal fats, this is where you want to prioritize spending your money. When a clean animal makes fat in its body, it stores the toxins there.[117] So, if that

---

[115] Teicholz, Nina. *The Big Fat Surprise: Why Butter, Meat and Cheese Belong in a Healthy Diet.* Paperback – January 6, 2015. Simon & Schuster; Reprint edition (January 6, 2015)

[116] https://www.ncbi.nlm.nih.gov/pmc/articles/PMC4424769/

[117] https://smile.amazon.com/Nourishing-Traditions-Challenges-Politically-Dictocrats-ebook/dp/B00276HAWG/ref=sr_1_1?crid=HJE2H3XFHSTK&keywords=nourishing+traditions+by+sally+fallon&qid=1663800316&s=-books&sprefix=nourishi%2Cstripbooks%2C169&sr=1-1

animal is being exposed to farm chemicals or given antibiotics and hormones, which are common practices in agriculture, then those things are going to be in its fat. This may shock you, but I agree with vegans who say that this is not what you want to be eating.

We raise our own cows and chickens, so I know exactly what they are eating and therefore, what I'm eating. That's how seriously I take this. The good news is that there are now online delivery companies and local stores where you can get grass-finished, organic animal fats and meats, which means you don't have to raise cows if you don't want to (although they are really cute!) These are the types of animal fats that you'll want to use for cooking with, not liquid oils, if at all possible.

It does not matter what the smoke point is on the bottle. Use saturated fats like lard (rendered pig fat), tallow (rendered cow fat), coconut oil, palm oil, butter, and heavy cream.

MEASURING YOUR INTAKE

You want to start with a high amount of fat so that you're not feeling tired—probably about 120 grams a day.[118] That's a lot of fat, and again, it has to be intentional because we are not used to putting that much fat on our food. Ideally, it is best to have a variety of different fats—just make sure they are high quality so that you don't create more inflammation while you are trying to reduce it because this will make up a large portion of your diet.

---

[118] https://smile.amazon.com/Whole-Soy-Story-Americas-Favorite/dp/0967089751/ref=sr_1_1?crid=I3L3DO5J1RJY&keywords=sally+fallon+soy&qid=1663800422&s=books&sprefix=sally+fallon+soy%2Cstripbooks%2C192&sr=1-1

The other components of a low insulin diet are protein and carbohydrates. It's good to have a variety of proteins, with the exception of soy. Soy is genetically modified and not usually properly fermented; therefore, the phytic acid is not deactivated and will bind to other nutrients in what you are eating, so that you don't get the nutrients in your expensive food. Additionally, it can really screw up your hormones in a big way. But go wild and enjoy other protein sources, including turkey, beef, lamb, mutton, chicken, elk, deer, quail, goose, duck, and so on. Your ideal amount of protein per day varies based on cancer status, activity level, gender, age, and so on, but generally you want around .75 to 1 gram per pound for an athletic individual or 0.4 grams per pound for those with cancer.[119]

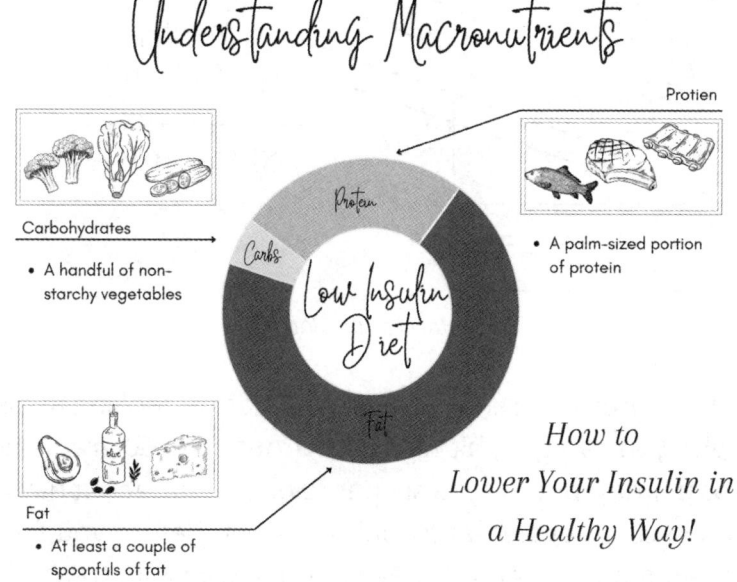

Figure 5-4: Understanding macronutrients

---

[119] https://www.wholesomeyum.com/how-to-calculate-net-carbs/

When it comes to carbs, I take into consideration where my clients are starting from and work them down to around 20-30 grams net carbs per day, spread out over the day. To determine how many carbs are in the food you're eating, subtract out any fiber, sugar alcohols, and allulose because those are not going to be digested by your body—this will give you your net carbs.

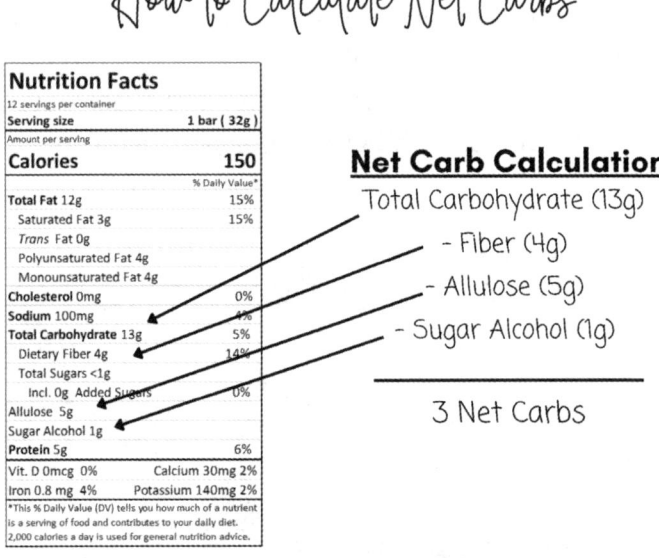

Figure 5-5: How to calculate net carbs

If you aren't currently in a disease state or looking to lose weight, you can go a bit higher to around 50-60 grams net carbs per day, but this is a slippery slope. Think about having just low carb veggies, and you'll do great. Before you freak out, remember—you can have a fun, low insulin treat with very few carbs if you are using things like almond or coconut flour and allulose, stevia, or monk fruit to sweeten it! Keep it clean though and avoid the artificial sweeteners.

Also, note that when you eat carbs, you get more insulin circulating, and if you're eating a lot of fat, it is going to be put into storage. That's the perfect storm for creating weight gain. Keep in mind, too, that this is a very bio-individual plan, and it's going to have a lot to do with things like your age, metabolic status, genetics, and activity level—they all play into how fast you burn fat.

Start with the guidelines above, but give yourself some grace. Once you get going, and you're feeling good and starting to see wins, then you can play with cycling out.[120] These are meals where you intentionally eat more carbs to keep your body metabolically flexible. I recommend eating sweet potatoes or plantains, not a Cinnabon washed down with a jug of orange juice.

What drives most people crazy in a low insulin diet is that they want to have it always be the same. Most of my clients just want me to tell them how to do it, and they'll follow the rules to the letter.

I'm going to give you a starting point, but I know that you don't want to have the same macros, the same foods, or the same eating schedule every day—you want to keep your body on its toes to create flexibility. This allows for a lot of wiggle room, and I have seen that, in the long run, this helps my clients because there's no stress if they screw up once in a while. But if you're falling off the wagon every single day and stopping at Dunkin' Donuts, then this is not going to work.

Keep in mind that there is a learning curve here, and that's why I said to give it three months to figure things out. Let your body have some time to adjust and find the kinds of foods you

---

[120] https://www.ncbi.nlm.nih.gov/pmc/articles/PMC5513193/#:~:text= Metabolic%20flexibility%20is%20the%20ability,obesity%20and%20 type%202%20diabetes.

like. I found that I don't always like low carb versions of my old favorites as much as I like new, creative ways of eating—I like thinking outside the box. You'll find all my favorite recipes in your private portal when you use the QR code at the end of the Introduction. So, get excited because there's good food coming that will make you feel amazing!

JAMIE'S CARB EPIPHANY

For Jamie, the first month was all about figuring out what she could eat. She tried to keto-ify her favorite treats and became frustrated because they weren't the same. We problem-solved, and I helped her learn how to bake, keto-style, and just eat differently. Even while she was still finding her footing, she started to lose weight, so she was encouraged to keep going.

In month two, Jamie started to dial in her macronutrients and realized that a lot of foods she was eating were higher in carbs than she'd thought. She also found that just because something claimed to be keto-friendly didn't mean it had enough fat for what she needed.

She then shifted into focusing on getting enough fat through sauces, salad dressings, and fat bombs (or high fat treats) to meet her needs. She soon found she was more satiated and lost even more weight. She was excited that she didn't have to starve while the weight slid off.

In the third month, Jamie realized that she was eating way more protein than she needed. She had inadvertently slipped into this habit and needed to bring her protein down to 75 grams per day so that her body wasn't converting it through gluconeogenesis into carbs. (This is exactly the pattern that I see most of my clients follow—they get the carbs out, get enough fat, then need to reduce their protein intake.)

Lo and behold, after the three months were over, Jamie said that she didn't miss the carbs as much as she had thought she would. She felt satiated and the food was yummy—she even found some fabulous treats so she didn't feel deprived! She was down 15 pounds and said she "finally felt comfortable" in her body.

Chapter 6
Problem-Solving with a Low Insulin Diet

During your transition to a low insulin diet, there are some potholes that may arise, and I want to give you six areas to keep your eye on. The first two are going to help prevent the problems that people sometimes have when lowering their insulin; the other four will help you customize the low insulin diet to your specific needs.

THE DILEMMA OF FAT DIGESTION

When you're eating more fats than your body is used to, you want to make sure that you can digest those fats—otherwise, they can make you very nauseous. This is a very common symptom that people have when lowering their insulin levels. Nausea due to problems digesting fat is tied into liver and gallbladder function.[121]

Doctors often say there's no real function for the gallbladder, but it is crucial to the emulsion (or breakdown) of the fats

---

[121] https://www.mdpi.com/2072-6643/12/2/540

you eat.[122,123] The liver makes bile, which not only helps you break down fats but is also a key mechanism to escort toxins out of your body.

The liver makes a steady flow of bile during the day and stores it in the gallbladder. When you eat a fatty meal, the gallbladder squirts the bile out into the small intestine to help you digest those fats so you can use them. If this process does not work properly, you excrete those precious fats and miss their benefits!

If you have had your gallbladder stolen (I mean removed), you'll want to make sure that you are doing some supplementation with fatty meals to encourage the digestion of fats without nausea.[124,125] I have yet to have a client come to me who has been told by the doctor who removed their gallbladder that this is necessary; they just tell them not to eat fats. This may solve the short-term problem of indigestion, but those fats are crucial for long-term health. (Remember how your cell membranes, hormones, and prostaglandins, and so on are made out of them?)

If you haven't been eating healthy fats in the needed quantities, it may startle your body to all of a sudden have a huge amount of them, so what I am about to suggest will help the transition as you teach your body what to do with them. I recommend bile support with things such as beets, coffee, green tea/matcha, ginger, curcumin, phosphatidylcholine (and regular choline), taurine, vitamin C, milk thistle, and dandelion

---

[122] https://www.hopkinsmedicine.org/news/media/releases/gallbladder_removal_is_common_but_is_it_necessary

[123] https://www.ncbi.nlm.nih.gov/books/NBK279386/#:~:text=The%20gallbladder%20stores%20and%20concentrates,and%20absorb%20fats%20from%20food.

[124] https://link.springer.com/chapter/10.1007/978-94-009-4904-1_2

[125] https://www.ncbi.nlm.nih.gov/pmc/articles/PMC1514056/

root. There are so many lovely supplements on the market that contain combos of these, and you can take some of them as a drink. (Recipes are available with the QR code at the end of the Introduction.)[126]

For those who do not have a gallbladder, you will need to take bile salt (or ox bile) at every meal when you are eating fats, which should be all of them. When you don't have a gallbladder, the bile the liver makes constantly drips out so that there is not a *whoosh* of it squeezed out when you have a meal. This means that there will be continual damage to the small intestine, since the bile is being released without food; therefore, gut healing is needed on an ongoing basis because the damage is continually occurring.[127]

Don't freak out, but my favorite way to get a backed-up gallbladder moving and healthy is through coffee enemas. When people can get over the "ick" factor, they actually come to me and tell me they like them (total parasympathetic Zen). I'm being serious here, so give it a try and let me know if you don't agree! (Use the QR code at the end of the Introduction for instructions.)

Coffee enemas work because the palmitic acid in coffee gets up into the liver through the hepatic portal vein and stimulates the release of bile. It helps clear out sluggish bile, break down any stones, and get the bile moving regularly.[128]

I have helped bring many clients back from the brink of needing their gallbladder removed. So, please don't feel that

---

[126] https://doi.org/10.1016/0378-8741(85)90009-1 ; https://doi.org/10.1039/c2fo30249g

[127] https://www.ncbi.nlm.nih.gov/books/NBK539902/

[128] https://draxe.com/health/coffee-enema/

you are a hopeless case here, no matter what your gallbladder status is—just take it slow and support the process proactively.

ELECTROLYTES AND THE KETO FLU

Not only does insulin prevent you from burning fat, it also messes with your electrolytes. This and fat digestion are behind the "keto flu" that some people get when they do keto without supporting the transition— so, now you won't have to deal with poor fat digestion or imbalanced electrolytes. When you eat carbohydrates, they cause you to produce insulin, which also signals your kidneys to retain sodium.[129] If you've ever dealt with any edema or water retention issues, this may be part of the issue.

When you don't have higher insulin levels, the kidneys are not getting signals to retain the sodium and will dump it, meaning you pee it out. This is not a bad thing, but it can disrupt how your body normally operates, especially if you aren't used to it.

If you don't transition slowly and gradually, you may need to supplement with electrolytes to keep your levels balanced. Otherwise, you may feel lightheaded, dizzy, headachy, or irritable. You may also have difficulty sleeping or with constipation, brain fog, or other issues.[130] These are all easily avoided by staying well hydrated and giving your body extra salt and electrolytes.

There are many great electrolyte drinks out there without sugars or artificial sweeteners. I like to get some with extra potassium, which is the one area that you might be deficient

---

[129] https://pubmed.ncbi.nlm.nih.gov/7028550/
[130] https://www.mayoclinic.org/diseases-conditions/hyponatremia/symptoms-causes/syc-20373711

in if you're eating a low insulin diet, as potassium is usually found in high carbohydrate foods, and it is almost impossible to get enough of. (My current favorite is Ultima. It comes in lots of fun flavors without a lot of unnecessary chemicals.)

This is also a good time to mention that it's important that you stay well hydrated. That means you should drink half your body weight in ounces every day—so, if you weigh 150 pounds, that means you should drink 75 ounces of water, which is about 2 to 3 quarts.[131]

Many of my clients think they're drinking enough liquids, but when I investigate, a lot of what they drink ends up being teas, coffee, and other diuretics. Diuretics will actually deplete your body of hydration. Anything with caffeine, sodas (diet and regular), alcohol, and packaged fruit juices will reduce your hydration status. (Sparkling water is not a diuretic.) If you are going to consume those, you want to make sure that you compensate by drinking even more water. When most of my clients realize this, they often decide to drink plain, filtered water because they don't want to drink that much liquid to compensate, but this is totally your choice.

Just a note—many people drink herbal teas thinking they're hydrating, and while they may be therapeutic, they can also be diuretics. Licorice tea is one that is not diuretic, is very healing for the adrenals, and tastes delicious!

THE SKINNY ON SWEETENERS

People who attempt a low insulin diet are often anxious that they're not going to be able to eat yummy treats. You will

---

[131] https://www.webmd.com/diet/features/water-for-weight-loss-diet#:~:text=%E2%80%9CIn%20general%2C%20you%20should%20try,ounces%20of%20water%20a%20day.

have to be more intentional and try some new recipes, but low carb baking can be amazing! There are many different kinds of healthy sweeteners that will allow you to have a fun treat without having the insulin spike.

You'll want to avoid sugar—honey, maple syrup, white sugar, brown sugar, coconut sugar, agave, rapadura, and high-fructose corn syrup—in any form. Even a "healthy" sugar won't be healthy for someone with blood sugar dysregulation. Artificial sweeteners like aspartame and sucralose are even worse because they are excitatory neuro-stimulators and are addictive.[132,133,134,135] I wouldn't touch those with a 10-foot pole, not even in chewing gum. (Don't worry—there are even some chewing gums like Spry and Pur that don't have these nasty toxins.)

> Even a "healthy" sugar won't be healthy for someone with blood sugar dysregulation.

When you are cooking, you'll want to choose healthy sweeteners such as stevia, allulose, monk fruit, or even some of the sugar alcohols, like erythritol and xylitol. Please note that some people are bothered by sugar alcohols, and some may have issues with stevia if ragweed is a problem for them—everyone's choice will be different.[136]

Of note—if you try stevia and don't like it, you're probably using too much. Sugar alcohols can also have a cold taste

---

[132] https://pubmed.ncbi.nlm.nih.gov/28198207/#:~:text=Aspartame%20(%CE%B1%2Daspartyl%2Dl,anxiety%2C%20depression%2C%20and%20insomnia.

[133] https://pubmed.ncbi.nlm.nih.gov/10882814/

[134] https://www.scientificamerican.com/article/artificial-sweeteners-confound-the-brain/

[135] Blaylock, Russell L., and Tom Weiner. *Excitotoxins: The Taste That Kills*. Blackstone Audio, Incorporated, 2011

[136] https://pubmed.ncbi.nlm.nih.gov/25449199/

afterward, which is why I prefer blends for baking. It is imperative to note that brands make a huge difference here, so try others if you have a bad experience—my favorite is Sweet Leaf's liquid flavors.

When my clients first start out, they want to try to recreate their old favorites. I am fine with this, as it is part of the adaptation process. Inevitably, they gradually make fewer attempts and find that they enjoy more foods that aren't re-creation of their old favorites. Instead, they enjoy new, outside-the-box creations.

Ideally, you'll want to use almond flour and coconut flour for baking because those are not going to have the carbohydrates and the insulin-spiking effect. (Don't be deceived by "gluten-free" items, which may still have plenty of carbs if they're made with other flours.) It's easy to get your hands on these items—they are available through Amazon, Costco, Walmart, and the like. Please know that these do not substitute for flour in recipes evenly—use recipes for these specifically. I'm excited by how many amazing treats come out daily that are already baked with these ingredients and without all the yucky preservatives!

As you refine your blood sugar dysregulation further, I also want to point out that stress can make your glucose go up as well. Whether you are having an argument with a spouse, or you have a deadline to meet, your body will release cortisol, which is a reaction to stress.[137,138] One of the things that cortisol does is to increase blood glucose levels. If you have a high-stress lifestyle, it's wise to take inventory and consider ways that you can reduce your stress levels, as this will go a long way to helping your low insulin diet.

---

[137] https://doi.org/10.1210%2Fjc.2010-0322
[138] https://doi.org/10.2188%2Fjea.JE20150183

BIO-INDIVIDUALITY AND FOOD SENSITIVITY

We've all heard people talking about food sensitivities and different things that they can't eat. I highly encourage you to recognize that this is a real issue. If you have any degree of leaky gut, partially digested food is getting into the bloodstream where it reacts with your immune system. The key to this is to make sure your food is completely digested, which we'll talk about in the upcoming gut section.[139]

In the meantime, if you have issues with nightshades, dairy, gluten, or other foods that irritate you, please continue to avoid those, but know that if you continue to do the healing work, you may not always have to avoid them.

For most people, healing the gut allows them to reintroduce these foods without problems.[140] If you just perpetually avoid them, more and more food sensitivities are usually created, as your body begins to react to other foods. Soon, you end up with a very restricted diet, which no one wants!

My client, Susie, was having a hard time with her food sensitivities. After a lot of digging, we discovered that it was microcrystalline cellulose in some of her supplements that caused her diarrhea. Once we removed that, things settled down quite a bit. So, please be aware that it may be something obscure that you're not thinking about, and you may want to utilize a practitioner to test you to identify what ingredient is bothering you. Just because a food is healthy for most people doesn't mean it's always good for you.

---

[139] https://www.ncbi.nlm.nih.gov/pmc/articles/PMC6893834/
[140] https://smile.amazon.com/Virgin-Diet-Drop-Foods-Pounds-ebook/dp/B00X3NIXFU/ref=sr_1_1?crid=II7B2USVMAHY&keywords=food+sensitivity+jj+virgin&qid=1663823856&s=books&sprefix=food+sensitivity+jj+virgin%2Cstripbooks%2C127&sr=1-1

It's All About Timing

I am so excited that intermittent fasting is getting more press because I am a huge fan of it and use it with many clients, but I don't suggest it for everyone. If you are hypoglycemic, you should NOT be doing any form of intermittent fasting. This will actually make your issues worse.

Symptoms of hypoglycemia come on before meals. They include feeling irritable, getting jittery or shaky, feeling light-headed, having poor energy before meals, and getting energized after meals.[141] If you have any of these symptoms, you should have a fat and protein snack between meals or a meal every two to three hours. As you go forward and have fewer of these symptoms, you can gradually stretch these times apart, eventually getting to three square meals a day.

Once you become a rock star at not snacking with no symptoms, then you can transition into intermittent fasting, which just means that you space out the time between your meals as much as possible—between dinner and breakfast the next day, for example.[142] Try to take a break from eating for twelve hours, then fourteen, then sixteen. By doing this, your period of eating during the day will become smaller and smaller. You still need to get all your nutrients in during that time, so you'll have quite large meals, and they may become closer together.

---

[141] https://www.mayoclinic.org/diseases-conditions/hypoglycemia/symptoms-causes/syc-20373685

[142] https://smile.amazon.com/Complete-Guide-Fasting-Jimmy-Moore-ebook/dp/B09PLL6VGN/ref=sr_1_1?crid=10Q7D3IL546AL&keywords=ultimate+guide+to+intermittent+fasting&qid=1663823955&s=books&sprefix=ultimate+guide+to+intermit%2Cstripbooks%2C147&sr=1-1

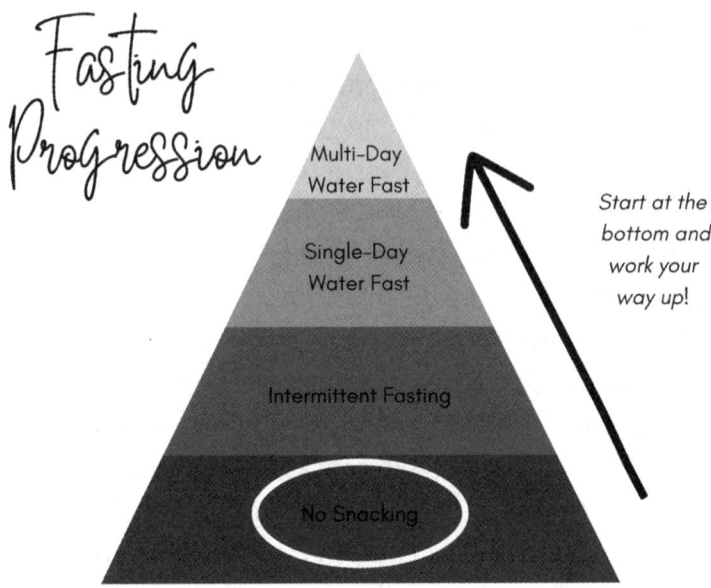

Figure 6-1: IT spectrum!

If you have questions about whether you are hypoglycemic or not, you can run a blood marker called *lactose dehydrogenase* (LD or LDH for short). If your blood work LDH is less than 140 U/L, then you'll want to keep your meals two to three hours apart. A note here—if you are already fat adapted (i.e., burning fat for fuel—you've been doing this a while already), you may show up as low LDH. You can clearly dismiss it if you don't have any symptoms of hypoglycemia.

THE IMPORTANCE OF FOOD QUALITY

There's a lot of dirty keto going on out there, and I want to prevent problems for you by stating something that is very important—quality matters. We talked about how animals store toxins in their fat, so it's important that you have organic fat. You want to eat clean, whole foods without a lot of additives, herbicides, preservatives, and chemicals because those are all going to inflame your body.[143] When you're trying to get inflammation under control, it makes no sense to be pouring gasoline on the fire of inflammation with these toxic chemicals.

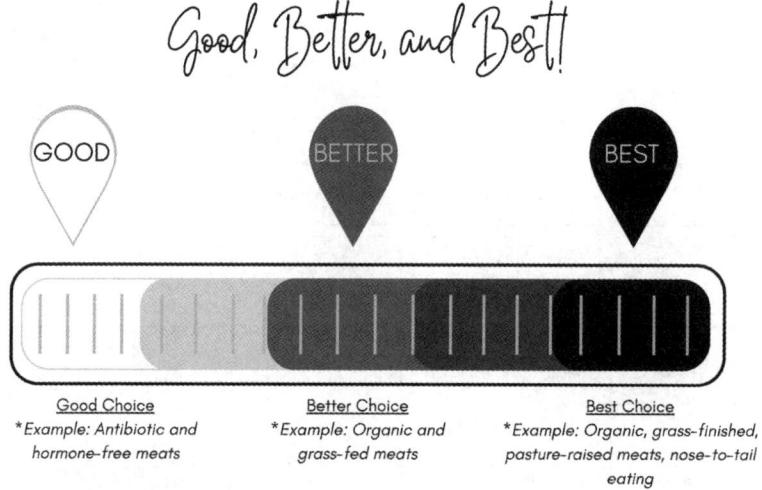

Figure 6-2: Good, better, best spectrum

I understand that everyone has a budget, so you're going to have to make choices on the good, better, best spectrum. That's why I gave you fats and meats as a priority. Do the best you can when choosing vegetables and fruits. Also, check out ewg.org, which lists the "Clean Fifteen" and the "Dirty Dozen" to help you prioritize your produce and reduce your exposure as much as possible to toxic chemicals.

---

[143] https://smile.amazon.com/Toxin-Solution-Products-Destroying-Health-ebook/dp/B01GCCT3D4/ref=sr_1_3?crid=3I2XI0UOZKSPZ&keywords=pizzorno&qid=1663862883&s=books&sprefix=pizzorno%2Cstripbooks%2C235&sr=1-3

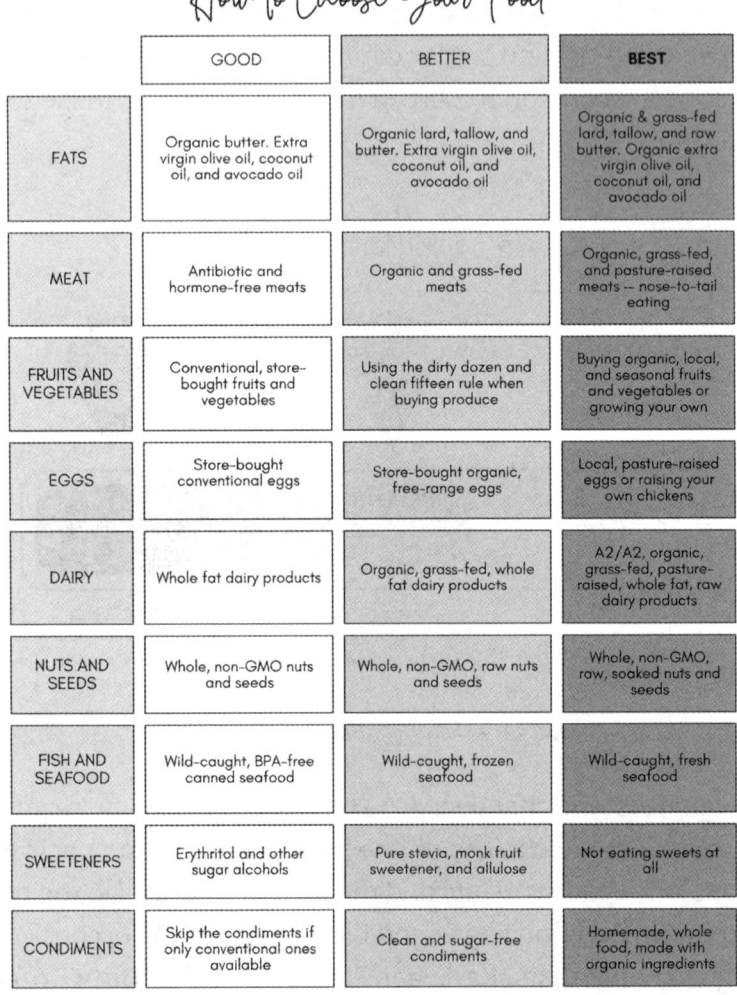

Figure 6-3: How to choose your food

Here are some personal examples—I do not eat zucchini unless it is organic because it is a GMO crop. I always make sure my berries are organic, but if it's something like an avocado, I will go ahead and get the non-organic form because it's not currently one of the most highly sprayed crops.

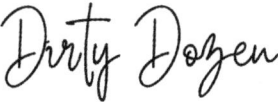 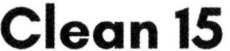

Dirty Dozen	Clean 15
1. Strawberries	1. Avocado
2. Spinach	2. Sweet Corn
3. Kale, Collard Greens, and Mustard Greens	3. Pineapple
4. Nectarines	4. Onions
5. Apples	5. Papaya
6. Grapes	6. Sweet Peas (Frozen)
7. Bell and Hot Peppers	7. Asparagus
8. Cherries	8. Honeydew Melon
9. Peaches	9. Kiwi
10. Pears	10. Cabbage
11. Celery	11. Mushroom
12. Tomatoes	12. Cantaloupe
	13. Mangos
	14. Watermelon
	15. Sweet Potatoes

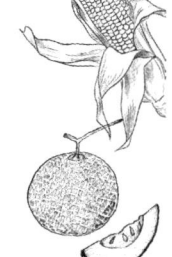
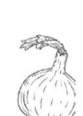
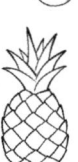
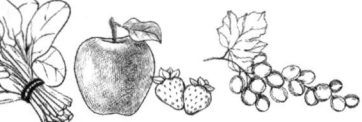

Figure 6-4: Dirty dozen and clean fifteen, currently

These ideals will allow you to personalize your low insulin diet (and your family's) and avoid possible pitfalls. These areas will shift with different seasons of life, being in a different environment, having different stress levels, and knowing the *why* behind what you're doing. In the big picture, listen to your body and adjust things according to your own needs.

Chapter 7
The Impact of Genetics

If being healthy and slim were just a matter of eating a low insulin diet, everyone would have robust health and look like a supermodel, right? Clearly, that is not all there is to the picture, and I'm not going to treat you as if you're stupid enough to think that way.

In the next chapters, I want to go through some specific areas that can screw up your body's functioning so that you'll know where to dig deeper. This discussion is also going to give you a bird's-eye view of all the areas that you need to focus on as you age.

I want to make sure that you don't feel crazy if some of these areas create havoc, hinder you from losing weight, and cause your joints to hold you back from living. In the bigger picture, I want you to understand that these "other factors" are going to play a huge part in—well, let's face it—how you die.

As I watch my father struggle with dementia, I am coming to a new understanding of how important quality of life is—it's not just about how old you live to be. It's just as important (if not *more* important) that you are mentally and physically capable until the end. I want to be able to play with my grandkids and remember all their names.

I feel like our society has gotten so off track with how we view health that we need a wake-up call—a clarification of what true health is and how we get back to it. Everyone needs to know that they have the power and ability to do what their body needs to feel good and live their most vibrant life.

I'll be honest with you—there are a lot of things that can work against your health. If you think these may be issues for you, you may need to do some further digging with a functional practitioner who can run the tests that I'm about to discuss. I hate reading books that point out a problem and leave you with no solution, so I am going to give you several things that you can do on your own that will allow you to clear out all the low-hanging fruit and see how much of an impact it makes.

Keep in mind that this is all very specific to you, and you likely won't have ALL of the things going wrong that I'm going to get into, but if you do, you will need to prioritize because there's still hope. Remember, most of my clients are folks with cancer, and I am blessed to see amazing recoveries. They are people, the same as you, who have similar things going wrong, just amplified.

How Much Do Your Genes Affect Your Health?

Health is a kaleidoscope of factors that all need to be in sync with each other in order to be harmonious. You'll want to look at every fragment to see if it works with the other pieces. When the pieces are off, you might be able to limp along and compensate, but if multiple pieces are off, that's where you get a perfect storm throwing you down the path toward chronic disease. If you understand what all of these factors are and keep your eye on them, you're going to be in a much better place to circumvent those chronic diseases and poor quality of life.

So many healthcare professionals look at disease as if it just happens by chance, or people say things like "Oh, I just have bad genetics." This is not the case if you understand all that goes into your health and what you can do to improve it—the reins are in your hands. Your genetics are simply the blueprint that God gave you to work with. When the contractor actually puts the house together, they can adjust the plans as needed, based on the materials that they have access to.

Epigenetics are the choices you make every day—for example, what you eat, what you drink, where you live, what you do, and how much you sleep—and how they affect your genes. Epigenetics have shown us that diet and lifestyle are more powerful than genetics alone because they will influence how the genes are actually expressed.[144] By making good diet and lifestyle choices, like going to bed at a reasonable hour and eating whole, unprocessed foods, you can choose the life you want. By making educated, self-disciplined choices every day, you can turn off chronic disease. You have the power.

I'm going to give you a little insight into my genetic profile to explain more. While I am able to look great in jeans (at least my husband says so), I don't have great genes. However, by understanding my genes, I have the tools to understand what is going to help me the most in terms of minimizing the bad genes and maximizing the good ones. I use a test that looks at the low penetrance genes, which are those that your diet,

---

[144] https://smile.amazon.com/Pottengers-Prophecy-Resets-Wellness-Illness/dp/1935052330/ref=sr_1_2?crid=2VT99UNIUV47H&keywords=pottenger&qid=1663864898&s=books&sprefix=pottenger%2Cstripbooks%2C182&sr=1-2

lifestyle, and supplements can impact in a huge way, then I use that to guide me into what food, lifestyle, and supplement choices I make every day.[145]

For example, I have what's called a *fast COMT genetic SNP* (single nucleotide polymorphism). SNPs are alterations from the more common DNA sequence variation that most people have.[146] In this case, it means that I tend to process my hormones and neurotransmitters super-fast; I just blow through them. This is good if I'm running high on my hormones—such as when I was estrogen dominant and had breast cancer. It actually helped me get my body back to where it could get the cancer into remission. However, on the other side of the coin, it works against me because I'm always low in neurotransmitters. So, this is an area that I need to strategically supplement with things like naturally occurring mineral lithium orotate to make sure that I feel good and that life is worth living.[147]

This is a great example of how gene variants are not necessarily good or bad, but they can have different effects on different people, depending on the combination or how they play out for you specifically. I know that drinking green tea (matcha) is imperative for me because it helps slow down my fast COMT, but for somebody else with a slow COMT, it may work against them by causing them to further slow their hormone processing and creating a hormone imbalance.[148]

---

[145] https://ascopubs.org/doi/abs/10.1200/jco.2000.18.11.2309
[146] https://smile.amazon.com/gp/product/0977636305/ref=ppx_yo_dt_b_search_asin_title?ie=UTF8&psc=1
[147] https://smile.amazon.com/Nutritional-Lithium-Cinderella-Mineral-Transforms-ebook/dp/B01FT4OGDI/ref=sr_1_1?crid=3CK6072PMOUXV&keywords=lithium+greenblatt&qid=1663865047&s=books&sprefix=lithium+greenblat%2Cstripbooks%2C185&sr=1-1
[148] https://aacrjournals.org/cancerres/article/63/21/7526/510667/Tea-Intake-COMT-Genotype-and-Breast-Cancer-in

That is not what you want, especially when you're talking about menopause symptoms or hormone-driven cancers.

I'm also blessed with some fabulous MTHFR genetic variants (notice the similarity to some words my kids aren't allowed to say), which means that I don't methylate well. *Methylation* is a fancy term describing hundreds of chemicals that your body transforms into other chemicals by adding a methyl group to them.[149] If you don't methylate well, that means that all sorts of processes in your body can slow to a grinding halt, depending on how backed up you are in a specific area. By supplementing strategically, most people can then get these processes back up and running appropriately, but you have to know to do this.

To know if you need supplementation, testing (usually blood work) can show you how your genes are expressing. I always keep an eye on my homocysteine levels, which gives me a real-time view of how my MTHFR genetics are actually playing out. If my homocysteine gets higher than seven, I will make sure that I am taking methyl B vitamins, especially robust levels of folate and B12 along with a little B5 and B6.[150,151] These levels need to be pretty high and in a methylated form to get my methylation going.

When I see a client's homocysteine come back high, that's when I want to run their genetics to see if this is something that they are just struggling with temporarily due to some kind of toxin exposure or if this is something that they are going to

---

[149] https://smile.amazon.com/Dirty-Genes-Breakthrough-Program-Optimize-ebook/dp/B072L4DSDC/ref=sr_1_1?crid=3SJ83GYJGRSI2&keywords=dirty+genes&qid=1663865015&s=books&sprefix=dirty+genes%2Cstripbooks%2C173&sr=1-1

[150] https://www.health.harvard.edu/staying-healthy/In_brief_B_vitamins_and_homocysteine

[151] https://www.ahajournals.org/doi/10.1161/01.str.0000198815.07315.68

need ongoing support with. The only way to know how you're doing is to test not only your genetics, but also how they are expressing epigenetically with bloodwork.

Looking at your genetics gives you the necessary info to direct and prioritize your choices, as well as insight into your weak links and what to do to strengthen them. Knowing your genetic predispositions is key, as is knowing the other areas that we're going to talk about in the next few chapters—your gut, your hormones (besides insulin), and the ever-expanding toxic soup that we live in.

Hold on tight—up next are some more hazards to watch out for.

Chapter 8
Go with Your Gut

Carla came to me sleep-deprived, confused, and in pain. She had been suffering from intense heartburn for months and was at her wit's end about what to do for it. Every night, she would have severe heartburn for several hours that would leave her writhing in agony. She was scared to eat anything in fear that it might bring on more pain. Only by sitting in weird positions and taking tons of antacids could she even get to sleep. She was popping Tums like candy and knew that something was very wrong.

Her doctor told her to go on proton pump inhibitor (PPI) medication, which would reduce her stomach acid, but she didn't want to be on medication for the rest of her life and had hope that there was some other way. I agreed there was.

We set about doing some upper gastric healing for the damage that had been done to her esophagus with the heartburn and slowly titrated up her levels of stomach acid. Lo and behold, the burning stopped once we got to a very high dosage. She was ecstatic, but I wasn't satisfied. Why did she need so much?

How the Digestive System Works

I'm going to start from the top because you always want to go top to bottom when addressing digestion.

> You always want to go top to bottom when addressing digestion.

Let's begin with the brain. Did you know that your thoughts before and during a meal will influence your digestion?[152] You want to be in a calm, *parasympathetic state* (the opposite of the fight or flight, or a *sympathetic state*) so that you can digest your food thoroughly.[153] When food enters your mouth and you start chewing, hormones and enzymes get activated to start digesting and preparing your body for what is going to happen. By thinking, smelling, and tasting sweet food, your body will actually release some insulin, which won't give you a huge spike, but it's good to know that this is occurring.[154]

After swallowing, the food gets to your stomach where it needs to be physically ground up further and chemically digested. The stomach should release *hydrochloric acid* (HCl) which lowers its pH to between 1.5 and 3.5.[155] This is significant because if the pH is not low enough, it's not possible to actually absorb the minerals you're eating.[156] While you may eat foods high in nutrients and take expensive supplements, you won't actually get any of them if your pH is not at a place to allow those minerals to be absorbed—you'll just have pricey pee.

---

[152] https://my.clevelandclinic.org/health/body/23266-parasympathetic-nervous-system-psns
[153] https://www.ncbi.nlm.nih.gov/pmc/articles/PMC7219460/
[154] https://pubmed.ncbi.nlm.nih.gov/25782410/#:~:text=Abstract,odor%20exposure%20may%20induce%20satiation.
[155] https://pubmed.ncbi.nlm.nih.gov/10421978/
[156] https://pubmed.ncbi.nlm.nih.gov/2543192/

Think about the implications of this in terms of the osteoporotic epidemic that we currently have—calcium is not absorbed if the pH isn't low enough. It makes me cringe every time we have a new client at our Pilates studio who has osteoporosis and is on PPI medications. Your doctor telling you to take some antacid when you're feeling heartburn does actually work in the moment, but it is not a good long-term solution.

Your stomach is like a blender. If you put your dinner in the blender, whiz it up, then let it sit on a warm windowsill with the lid still firmly attached, what would happen after several hours? The carbohydrates that you ate would start to ferment, which would eventually pop the lid right off.

That's basically what happens in your stomach. When you don't have enough HCl secreted, the food can't be broken down properly—it ferments and forms gasses. The valve that holds the food in your stomach and out of your esophagus then pops open, and you'll burp. Sometimes, the food can even be pushed up into the esophagus, which is what causes the heartburn feeling. While the stomach is designed to hold very acidic contents, the esophagus is not.

You should also know that the food in the stomach is released into the small intestines by a special valve, and the secret handshake to get through is having a low enough pH. But wait—it gets better! Not only does having your stomach pH low help your body to break down food, but it also acts as an acid wash for any pathogens that would get into your body via your food.[157]

Four women go into a sushi bar (no, this isn't the setup for a bad joke). They all share the same sushi, which is

---

[157] https://www.ncbi.nlm.nih.gov/pmc/articles/PMC2223456/

contaminated by some nasty *E. coli* bacteria. Three of them end up with food poisoning. The other has no problem with the sushi and feels great. What's the difference among these four women?

The woman who didn't get sick had enough stomach acid to effectively kill the pathogens that were in the sushi, while the others didn't. Which woman do you want to be? (And just so you know, I never go for sushi without my HCl!)

The tricky thing is that there is not a convenient test to see what your stomach pH is. But have no fear! I'm giving you the instructions on how to do the HCl challenge to determine your levels. This process allows you to ramp up your HCl levels very, very slowly so you can feel when you get your maximum tolerated dosage and not overshoot the moon and give yourself heartburn.

See, there's only so low (i.e., the bottom range) that you want your stomach acid level to be, and you'll know that you've found it because it will give you heartburn or other digestive discomfort. That's where you back off a little and repeat at every meal. This process is a little tricky, and I'll talk you through all the details when you use the QR code found at the end of the Introduction.

Signs You Are Not Producing Enough Stomach Acid
(hypochlorhydria)

- Heartburn / Indigestion
- Acid Reflux / GERD
- Brittle hair and peeling nails
- Protein doesn't sound appealing or taste good
- Feeling unusually full after even a small meal
- Burping after meals
- Bloating after meals
- Constipation or diarrhea
- Nausea when taking supplements
- Flatulence
- Undigested food in stool

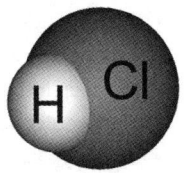

8-1.a Signs you are not producing enough stomach acid

Consequences of Hypochlorhydria
(low stomach acid / HCl)

- Your minerals and certain vitamins don't get absorbed, which leads to deficiency diseases such as osteoporosis, anemia, and others

- Pepsin doesn't get activated — protein doesn't get broken down and therefore doesn't taste good to you

- Reflux, GERD, heartburn

- First line of defense is gone — bacteria, viruses, parasites, and the like are not killed and are allowed to get into the gut

- H. pylori can overgrow in stomach — gastric cancer

- Other digestive juices don't get stimulated — bile, pancreatic enzymes, CCK, bicarbonate, and so on

HCl should make the pH in your stomach 1-3

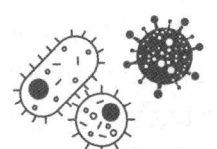

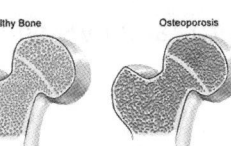

8-1.b Consequences of hypochlorhydria

Nutritional Pilates | 127

Why Don't I Have Enough Stomach Acid?

Factors that lower HCl:
- *Dehydration*
- *Stress*
- *Medications*
- *Zinc deficiency*
- *Sluggish bile flow*
- *Hiatal hernia*
- *Thyroid issues*
- *B vitamin deficiency*
- *Age (lower with age)*
- *H. pylori* infection
- *Excess alcohol consumption*
- *Surgery of the stomach*

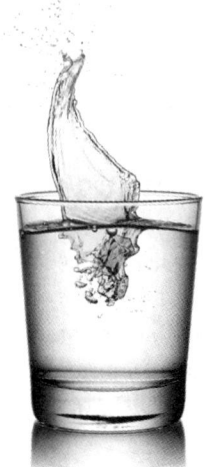

8-1.c Why don't I have enough stomach acid?

Figures 8-1.a.b.c: Roles of HCl

At this point, you may be asking what would cause your stomach acid to not be low enough—the two biggest reasons are dehydration and stress. (Anybody else see that these might be issues with most Americans?) There are also some other nutrients that are needed for the process, such as B6 and zinc.[158] How ironic that a mineral (zinc) is needed to help your body absorb minerals, so when you don't have it, you can't get it.

HCl is not a sexy supplement—the clouds don't part with rainbows shooting out of them when you start taking it. However, it is the lynchpin in making sure that food gets

---

[158] https://smile.amazon.com/Why-Stomach-Acid-Good-You-ebook/dp/B00AE1M1R0/ref=sr_1_1?crid=39IMEMHCNUF3W&keywords=why+you+want+stomach+acid+wright&qid=1663866125&s=books&sprefix=why+you+want+stomach+acid+wright%2Cstripbooks%2C159&sr=1-1

digested, you absorb all those nutrients, and you kill any possible pathogens that come into your body through your food. Yet, the conventional Western standard of care wants us to do the opposite.[159] When I go into Costco and see the massive displays of Prilosec, it makes me a little crazy. The only thing that keeps me from screaming and throwing the boxes all over the place is that it would embarrass my poor teenage daughters.

But it also makes me sad because I know how many people are going to have issues from this medication, and no one is going to connect the dots for them so they can make a different choice.

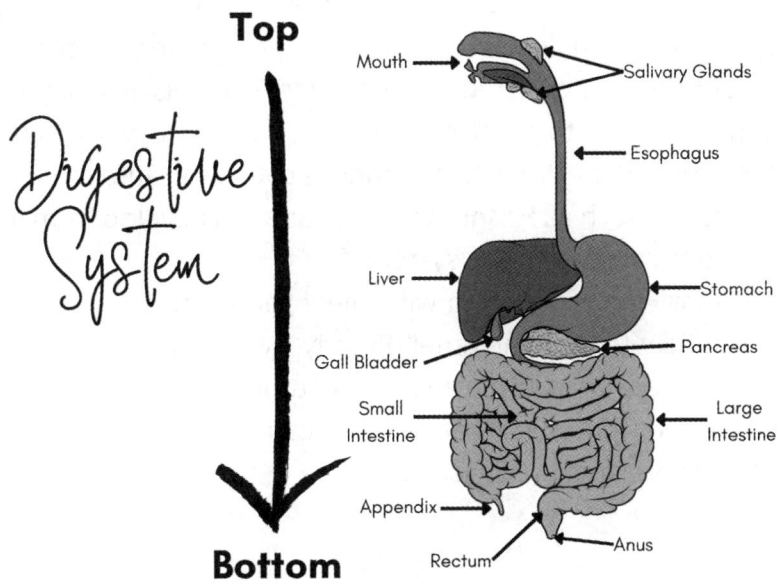

Figure 8-2: Digestive system

---

[159] https://www.ncbi.nlm.nih.gov/pmc/articles/PMC7828248/

All right, back to our digestive system—so the food gets down into the small intestines. There, it gets a nice alkaline wash to shift that pH higher. Then, because of the low pH, the digestive enzymes are released by the pancreas, and bile is released from the gallbladder to continue the digestion process as the food winds through your system. (We already discussed how critical bile is; you want that to be released!)

The small intestines are where nutrient absorption should occur, but one of the biggest problems here is that the small intestine can be leaky. Usually, the single cell layer of the intestines is only one cell thick, but the cells are squished together pretty tightly so that only super-small, broken-down molecules can get into the bloodstream for distribution throughout the body. But when these cells separate, then larger, partially digested food molecules can get through.[160,161] In your bloodstream, these undigested food particles set off alarms for your immune system to attack because they do not recognize these foreign invaders. When this continues over time, autoimmune conditions such as Hashimoto's disease can develop from an overstimulated immune system.[162,163]

What I get most often with client food sensitivity panels is "But I eat that all the time!" Exactly—your immune system is targeting that food because it is getting through your leaky gut in a not fully digested state and causing an attack, which is what your body should do.[164]

---

[160] https://www.ncbi.nlm.nih.gov/pmc/articles/PMC7828248/
[161] https://gut.bmj.com/content/68/8/1516.abstract
[162] https://www.frontiersin.org/articles/10.3389/fimmu.2017.00598/full?furriel=99b129e5a1ffa09775e93a4de7a4f2eab9269be1
[163] https://link.springer.com/article/10.1007/s12016-011-8291-x
[164] https://www.ncbi.nlm.nih.gov/pmc/articles/PMC1417187/

The solution is threefold:

1. Make sure you're digesting your food completely.
2. Do some healing work to make sure the junctions are tight, and there's no leaky gut.
3. Make sure to address whatever pathogens or toxins were making your gut leaky in the first place.

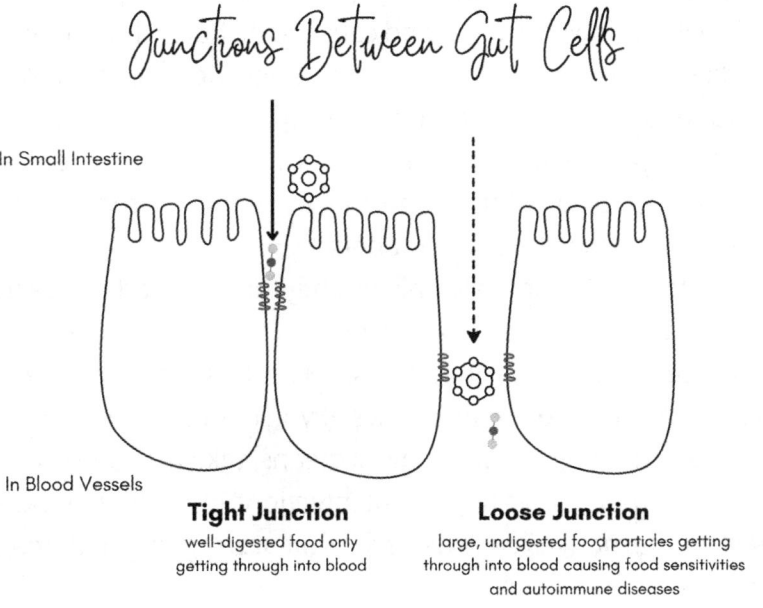

Figure 8-3: Tight junctions

In order to make sure that you are digesting your food completely, you will want to start with the HCl challenge, as that is the first domino in the domino train that you need to get your digestion rolling.

Doing the Healing Work

I recommend foods like homemade bone broth, aloe vera, and short-chain fatty acids, along with herbs and nutrients to heal your gut, and to get to the root cause, you'll want to look at your stool for potential pathogens such as parasites as well as chemicals you may be ingesting.[165,166,167,168]

Chemicals such as NSAIDs (non-steroidal anti-inflammatory medications), antibiotics, and glyphosate are the top offenders in breaking down your gut and causing the holes that allow the undigested food into your blood.[169] Over the counter NSAIDs include ibuprofen, naproxen, and aspirin (brand names you might recognize are Advil, Motrin, Aleve, Ascriptin, Bayer, and Ecotrin) are also culprits, and there are many others with a prescription, so check your labels.[170]

As for antibiotics, not only do they kill the good gut bacteria (which we'll get to in a second), but they also do serious damage to your small intestines.[171] I understand that there is a time and a place for antibiotics. If you're in the hospital with a life-threatening infection, by all means, take them. However, there are many ways to prevent infections in the first place, as well as alternatives such as herbs that aren't going to damage your gut.

---

[165] https://www.ncbi.nlm.nih.gov/pmc/articles/PMC2887640/
[166] https://www.mdpi.com/1422-0067/18/5/1051
[167] https://gut.bmj.com/content/35/1_Suppl/S35.abstract
[168] https://www.ncbi.nlm.nih.gov/pmc/articles/PMC6121872/
[169] Seneff, Stephanie. *Toxic Legacy: How the Weedkiller Glyphosate Is Destroying Our Health and the Environment*, (Chelsea Green Publishing, 2021).
[170] https://www.ncbi.nlm.nih.gov/pmc/articles/PMC7426480/#:~:text=NSAID%2Dinduced%20toxicity%20in%20the,anemia%2C%20strictures%2C%20and%20ulcerations.
[171] https://www.ncbi.nlm.nih.gov/pmc/articles/PMC5725362/

We have less and less ability to choose whether we are exposing ourselves to toxic chemicals. Herbicides are incredibly frustrating—I can see how much damage they do in my clients.[172] It is very hard to know if what you are eating has glyphosate on it or if it is genetically modified (GMO), so try and reduce your levels of toxins by eating organic as much as possible.

Here's the good news—when you go on a low insulin diet, you are going to eliminate a huge percentage of the foods that have glyphosate on them. So, you're already on the right path, even if you don't get everything organic just by not eating carbohydrates—these are crops that are the most heavily sprayed and contaminated.

THE END OF THE DIGESTIVE JOURNEY

After food travels through the small intestines, it goes into the colon (aka the large intestine), which is where your gut microbiome resides. All the good bacteria that you're hearing so much about will chow down on the food that has not been digested and absorbed in the small intestines, which is all the soluble and insoluble fibers. These are food for your good bacteria.

Being the altruistic critters that they are, they will actually make things like short-chain fatty acids, vitamin K, and B vitamins.[173] We're learning more every day on how helpful these gut bacteria are and all the wonderful things they do for us. To show our appreciation, we want to make sure that we

---

[172] https://www.ncbi.nlm.nih.gov/pmc/articles/PMC3945755/
[173] LeBlanc, Jean Guy, Florian Chain, Rebeca Martín, Luis G. Bermúdez-Humarán, Stéphanie Courau, and Philippe Langella. "Beneficial effects on host energy metabolism of short-chain fatty acids and vitamins produced by commensal and probiotic bacteria." *Microbial cell factories* 16, no. 1 (2017): 1–10.

give them everything they need to thrive, and we've come to learn that their favorite treats are fibers known as prebiotics found in foods such as dandelion greens, garlic, leeks, chicory, Jerusalem artichokes, inulin, acacia, and onions, among others.[174,175]

I have an amazing way to get a whole food fiber source with excellent diversity. Using the QR code at the end of the Introduction, take a look at the Green Shot there and show your appreciation to your gut microbiome.

Things like parasites, dysbiotic bacteria, or yeast overgrowth can also reside in the colon. You can often connect them to symptoms you may be having, like bloating, gas, GI discomfort and pain, cravings, skin eruptions, brain fog, deficiencies, and so on. If you have been eating a high carb diet for a significant period of time or have taken antibiotics, yeast will usually become overgrown. In fact, one of the immediate reactions to antibiotics is to have a backlash of yeast.[176] I mention this specifically because yeast will create cravings for carbohydrates because that's what yeast likes to eat.

If you are having a hard time with a low insulin diet in terms of craving carbohydrates, the answer is to do the low insulin diet. Over time, this way of eating will help you move past those cravings. However, you may need additional help addressing the possible yeast overgrowth driving them.[177] There's a great yeast culture test that also shows exactly what herbs will be most effective at getting it under control.

---

[174] https://www.webmd.com/diet/foods-high-in-prebiotic#1
[175] https://www.ncbi.nlm.nih.gov/pmc/articles/PMC7468733/
[176] https://www.healthline.com/health/yeast-infection-from-antibiotics#_noHeaderPrefixedContent
[177] https://www.cellphysiolbiochem.com/Articles/000139/

As the food exits the body, I want to make sure that you know what your poop should look like. This will give you some great information on what's going on, especially when things are going wrong. If your poop is floating, light colored, or greasy looking, and you have nausea, these might be indicators that you're not digesting fat properly.[178] If there's undigested food particles that you're seeing in your poop, make sure you're getting HCl to kickstart the domino train of digestion.

If you are constipated or have diarrhea, that's an indication that your transit time is not appropriate, and there may be some issues to look at in terms of hydration, thyroid function, and pathogens.[179,180]

Ideally, everyone should have more than one bowel movement per day (seriously). The gastrocolic reflex increases colon contractions, which cause you to poop in reaction to your stomach stretching when you eat. You can see this in babies who, when they eat or nurse, will poop almost immediately.[181] When we get stressed, dehydrated, or have pathogens or thyroid imbalance, our timing becomes off.[182]

If you're not having at least one bowel movement a day, you can take higher doses of magnesium or vitamin C or drink senna tea to help clear things out, but these are not long-term solutions. Make sure that you dig deeper because there's a reason your stool isn't right, and you want to make sure that reason is addressed.

---

[178] https://www.cellphysiolbiochem.com/Articles/000139/
[179] https://www.ncbi.nlm.nih.gov/pmc/articles/PMC5872693/
[180] https://pubmed.ncbi.nlm.nih.gov/2070959/
[181] https://www.babycareadvice.com/blogs/development/infant-reflexes
[182] https://www.ncbi.nlm.nih.gov/pmc/articles/PMC2699000/

Remember, every weird symptom that you have is your body's way of trying to communicate something to you, so learn to listen to it. If you pay attention to your symptoms, you can then learn how to address the root causes and support your body so it can really shine.

> *"All disease begins in the gut."*
> — **HIPPOCRATES**

A Client's Digestion Is Back on Track

My hope is that by getting your gut in a healthy place and having enough HCl, you can avoid a lot of these chronic diseases, just like Carla did. She did some gut testing and found that she had an *H. pylori* infection, which can cause heartburn by destroying the cells that make stomach acid. She addressed the *H. pylori*, and her need for HCl was drastically reduced.

H. pylori infections can lead to stomach and intestinal cancer. Not having enough HCl over time can lead to all sorts of deficiency issues, like osteoporosis and leaky gut, which also can lead to autoimmune conditions. None of this was on Carla's radar—she just wanted to be out of the immediate pain. Not only did she feel better, but she became more energetic, her brain got clearer, and her quality of life went through the roof. She is now sleeping through the night and waking up refreshed. She stopped worrying about what she could and couldn't eat and enjoys time with her family once again.

Chapter 9
Hormones

Olivia came to me because she had about 30 pounds to lose. She was tired, feeling run-down, and incredibly frustrated. She had tried lots of different diets, including a paleo diet, bone broth diet, and keto diet. She also exercised regularly but hadn't really seen anything shift. Oftentimes, there are some other factors that can block weight loss, so we decided to start with a comprehensive blood panel to see what was going on.

Her thyroid-stimulating hormone (TSH) came back at 4.3—this is technically within the lab range, which is created by taking the average results of all their clients plus two standard deviations, but it wasn't where I knew she'd feel good. The lab range has nothing to do with how people actually feel—it's simply an average of sick people's results.[183,184]

When I'm looking at labs, the functional range I use is based on where people are healthy and feeling good. For the TSH, I want it to be between one and two, preferably closer

---

[183] https://www.rupahealth.com/post/how-functional-medicine-provider-look-at-optimal-lab-ranges
[184] https://www.testing.com/articles/laboratory-test-reference-ranges/

to one. Olivia's insulin was also high, at 13.4—I like this to be below eight, if not lower.

Here we had two smoking guns—her blood sugar and insulin were dysregulated. We had a long discussion, and I explained that there could be some other things that were blocking her from progressing. We agreed to start by just working on diet and thyroid support and see how much that shifted things before diving into more extensive testing.

How the Thyroid Works

The thyroid has a whole communication system, or negative feedback loop, that continually monitors what the body needs and provides appropriate support.[185] The hypothalamus, which is in your brain, senses how much thyroid hormone is in circulation and sends a signal to the pituitary gland right below it. The pituitary is then tasked with sending out a hormone called TSH (thyroid-stimulating hormone) to the thyroid to tell it how much more it needs to make and put into circulation.

The thyroid, which is a butterfly-shaped gland in the front of your neck, then makes the actual thyroid hormone—predominantly in the inactive form (T4), but there's also a little of the active form (T3). These hormones go into the bloodstream where they attach to a protein, kind of like how you have to be in a car if you're on the highway. They circulate around the body, and when it needs more active thyroid hormone, the liver activates the T4 into T3. (This can also be done somewhat in the gut and in some other areas.)

---

[185] https://smile.amazon.com/Still-Thyroid-Symptoms-Tests-Normal-ebook/dp/B00A3K01Q6/ref=sr_1_1?crid=3L5UY7TR565OR&keywords=datis+thyroid&qid=1663875216&s=books&sprefix=datis+thyroid%2Cstripbooks%2C238&sr=1-1

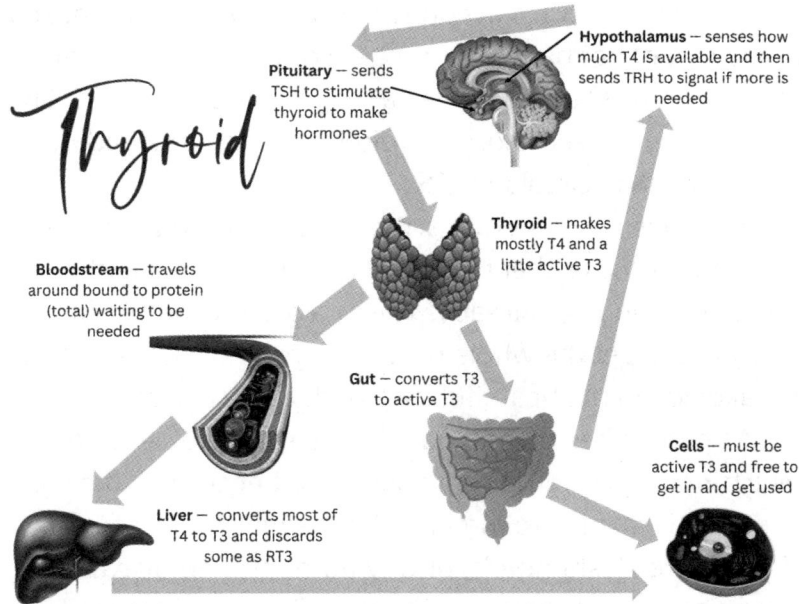

Figure 9-1: Thyroid feedback loop

When the liver senses that there is too much T4, it will discard some of it by converting it into reverse T3 (RT3). While the active T3 is circulating around in the bloodstream, it is able to be taken out of its "car" and used by any of the cells in the body as needed. It just has to enter the cell to be put to use, although there are some possible blockers.

I hope this gives you a better picture of the complexity of the thyroid hormone and how there are so many beautiful mechanisms designed to create a powerful, self-regulating negative feedback loop. All of this must be very precise because the thyroid hormone controls the body's energy production, and when there's not enough of it, nothing works quite right.

Today's standard of care just looks at the TSH, which was high in Olivia's case. It's like the pituitary is screaming at the thyroid, "Make more hormone now!" However, when I looked at the rest of her panel (because we ran all of the markers), I could see that she actually had a slightly elevated free T3. She didn't actually need more thyroid hormone—she had more than enough in circulation.[186]

Why was Olivia's brain screaming at her to make more hormone? It was either normal or elevated, meaning she had more than enough already. This is a great example of why you want to get the whole picture so you can see where the breakdown in the beautiful loop of thyroid regulation lies.

As part of her thyroid panel, I tested Olivia's antibodies, which would give me insight about whether she had the most common form of autoimmune disease, which is Hashimoto's. If you have Hashimoto's, or any autoimmune disease, it is imperative to support the organ that's being attacked by your own body, but you also must address the immune system that's doing the attacking and calm it down in order to get things into remission. That's the part of the equation that is not happening with today's standard of care because typically only the TSH is run.

If you have Hashimoto's, you need to completely shift what you should be eating and supplementing. With a sluggish thyroid (no antibodies and high TSH), you might want to take some iodine because it is the building block for thyroid hormones (literally—the numbers 3 and 4 in T3 and T4 are the numbers of iodine molecules).

However, if you have Hashimoto's with elevated thyroid antibodies, taking iodine is like pouring gasoline on an immune

---

[186] https://www.sciencedirect.com/science/article/abs/pii/S0025619612606946

system fire.[187] Even if the person needs iodine desperately, they're going to intensify the attack on the thyroid and ultimately, cause the quick destruction of that gland.[188] In no situation would I give somebody with Hashimoto's iodine, and I get very specific about making sure that there's no level of iodine in any of the supplements they take because it is common in many supplements. The individual also must be gluten-free, as gluten will also speed up the destruction of the thyroid.

To get Olivia's insulin down, she switched to a low insulin diet. She was already eating clean, whole foods, so it was really about finding low insulin treats, so she could really dial it in. Since all the hormones are downstream from insulin, this also helps with supporting thyroid function.

In terms of supplements, instead of giving her a thyroid glandular, like she would typically get with a high TSH, she took phosphatidylserine, which is support for her brain, where the real problem was at.

I just got her retest back and was excited to see that her TSH is now 2.65 and her insulin is at 7.6! While her TSH could come down a little further, her insulin looks lovely, and the good news is, she's already lost 15 pounds, which is halfway to her goal weight. Best of all, she's feeling more energized and has clearer mental capacity.

Hopefully, you can see here that it's not one-size-fits-all when looking at thyroid hormones. If I had just seen her TSH, I would have wanted to give her a thyroid glandular, which would not have addressed the issue.

---

[187] Wentz, Izabella, *Hashimoto's Protocol: A 90-Day Plan for Reversing Thyroid Symptoms and Getting Your Life Back.* HarperCollins, 2020.
[188] https://www.sciencedirect.com/science/article/abs/pii/S1568997201000167

List of Thyroid Markers to Ask For:

- TSH
- T4, free
- T3, free
- T4, total
- T3, total
- Reverse T3
- TGB antibodies
- TPO antibodies

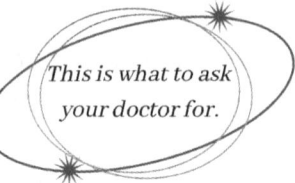

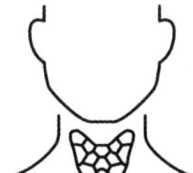

Figure 9-2: Thyroid markers to ask for

CORTISOL, SLEEP, AND STRESS

Michelle wanted to reverse her osteoporosis. She is a petite woman and was afraid of falling and shattering bones. This was making her cautious and scared when she and her husband went hiking together. She was a Pilates client, so I knew she was already educated and doing the right movements for osteoporosis, but there was something else going on. She was also having gas after meals, chronic headaches, sugar cravings, and trouble sleeping through the night, which was causing her to be irritable and not functioning well throughout the day.

Michelle was on a plant-based diet when we first started working together, so we discussed adding in some animal products, as they are more bioavailable. She also started the HCl challenge to make sure she was digesting her food properly, especially meat and minerals.

I recommended that she use her spit or urine (not blood) in a hormone panel to see what else might be throwing her body off, as there are many reasons that she would be losing bone mass. Her sex hormones were great, but when we looked at her adrenal hormones, we found her cortisol levels were through the roof—they were five times what they should have been!

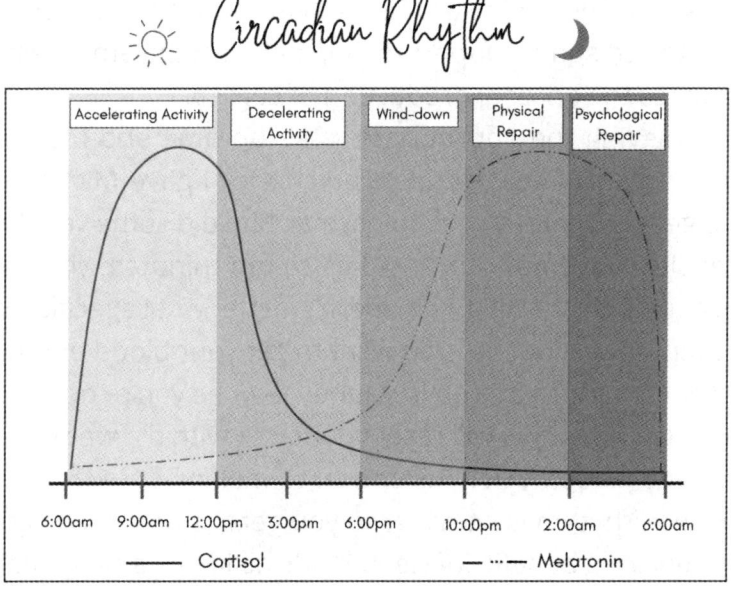

Figure 9-3: Circadian rhythm

The circadian rhythm is the dance that your hormones (cortisol and melatonin) do to keep you asleep at the right time and wake you up at the right time.[189] Cortisol can also be thrown off balance when you're under a lot of stress. It can derail the body's process for constant bone remodeling, which

---

[189] https://nigms.nih.gov/education/fact-sheets/Pages/circadian-rhythms.aspx#:~:text=Circadian%20rhythms%20are%20physical%2C%20mental,the%20study%20of%20circadian%20rhythms.

is where old bone is demolished and new bone is laid down.[190] When the demolition process is faster than the rebuilding process, you have osteoporosis.

Michelle started a low insulin diet to make sure that her hormones as a whole were working well together. She also did the HCl challenge and discovered that she was not making any stomach acid at all, which would explain why she felt she couldn't digest meat well. I recommended some adaptogenic herbs, specifically for calming down her high cortisol. She also started some support to help her hypothalamus, which regulates the adrenal production of cortisol.

Achieving the appropriate wake-up time and resetting your cortisol is key. Here's a quick trick I gave Michelle to help get her pattern back to normal. She did some very high intensity movement for just five to ten minutes when she woke up each morning.[191] It doesn't matter what specific form of exercise you do, but you want to get your blood pumping and get the morning sun in your eyes while you're doing it, if possible. Doing this will reset your clock within a week or so.

Good sleep hygiene is critical to making sure that your circadian rhythm is working, so you get the full rejuvenating and repairing benefits of sleep.[192] Michelle had a sleep makeover that included making her room completely dark, getting all the electronic devices out, lowering the temperature of the room, making sure her bedtime was reasonable, and limiting blue light and screen time for a couple of hours before bed.

---

[190] https://www.acpjournals.org/doi/abs/10.7326/0003-4819-147-8-200710160-00006
[191] https://doi.org/10.1016%2Fj.tips.2013.09.002
[192] https://www.thieme-connect.com/products/ejournals/abstract/10.1055/a-0905-3103

But the biggest area of change for Michelle was the intangible stress management. As she and I talked, it was clear that stress was a very big part of her life, and it was the challenging part of getting this under her control—she is always on the go-go-go and didn't see a need to slow down. We took things one step at a time, and when we retested six months later, her cortisol had come down to almost within range.

She was sleeping through the night, she had no more gas and bloating, she enjoyed animal protein, her energy had improved, she had lost her sugar cravings, and her headaches had even disappeared. Her osteoporosis wouldn't have resolved that quickly, but she was excited with the progress and now had hope she could put it in remission.

The hardest part for Michelle was slowing down, but she was a strong woman who was determined to feel her best. She now had tools to assess, manage, and maintain her stress levels, and it has paid off for her big time because now she knows how to feel good and what to do to stay that way.

The Process for Regulating Sex Hormones

Kaylea and her husband came to me when they were ready to conceive their third child. They already had two beautiful daughters, but she had had trouble conceiving the last one due to polycystic ovarian syndrome (PCOS). She wanted to avoid some of the heartache of unsuccessfully trying to conceive or of losing babies through miscarriages, and she knew that there were some diet components of PCOS that she needed to address.

She brought her husband with her to see me because she wanted to make sure that he heard all this, as he was not excited about making any changes to his standard American diet, and she knew herself well enough to know that if he was eating junk, she'd also be eating it. However, she and her husband were willing and open to doing anything to have more precious little babies.

That there are any babies born at all is astonishing to me. The complex dance that our female sex hormones do to make babies is a complete miracle, to say nothing of sperm development.

Let me start out by emphasizing that female sex hormones, as well as the cortisol we just discussed, are all made out of cholesterol by the body. If you don't have enough cholesterol, that's going to be a problem.[193] The first day of a woman's period is what we consider to be the beginning of a new cycle. This is when the follicle stimulating hormone (FSH) is sent down from the brain to the follicles developing in the ovaries. Each month, there is a development race where seven or eight follicles compete to see who is the strongest and can create the most estrogen. The winner gets crowned the dominant follicle and is the one that gets the opportunity to become a baby.

---

[193] https://www.ncbi.nlm.nih.gov/pmc/articles/PMC3636985/

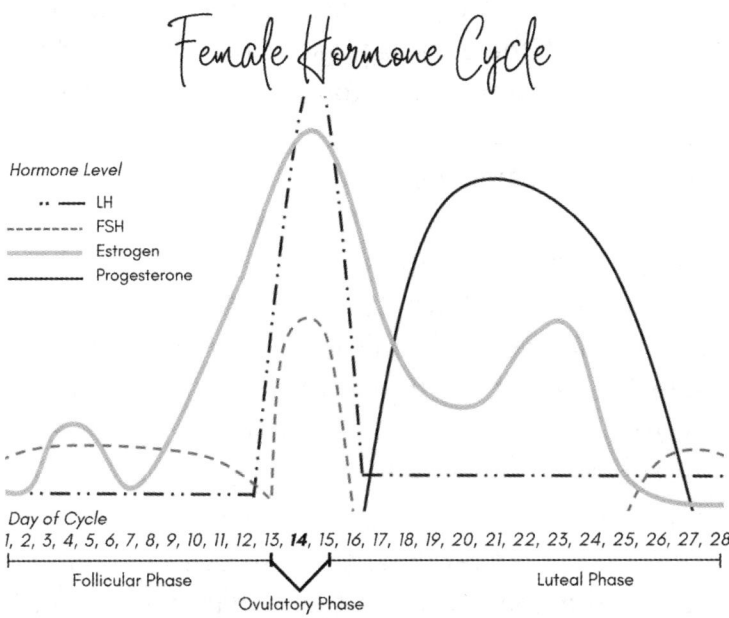

Figure 9-4: Female hormone cycle

At the end of the contest, the spike of estrogen signals the luteinizing hormone (LH) to be released by the brain. One of the things the LH does is to release proteolytic enzymes that eat a hole in the dominant follicle so that the egg can escape. While the egg is making its way down the fallopian tubes into the uterus, praying that it gets to meet a cute sperm, the follicle develops into what's called the *corpus luteum,* which becomes its own endocrine gland and makes the progesterone.[194] This is what is going to help to thicken the lining of the uterus and prepare everything for a nice, healthy pregnancy. It's kind of like decorating a baby's nursery.

Now, if an egg should meet its soulmate sperm and get fertilized, then a message is sent back to the corpus luteum

---

[194] https://www.ncbi.nlm.nih.gov/books/NBK279054/

to continue to make progesterone so the pregnancy will hold and be healthy. If the poor egg is still single at the end of the month, the corpus luteum will stop making progesterone, and that is what will start to stimulate the whole cycle over again, starting with the sloughing off of the lining of the uterus in the form of a period.

That's a pretty complicated dance of hormones. If you think back over what I just described, it all begins with the health of that follicle before any of this starts. So, what is going to create that perfect, healthy egg? It's a nutrient-dense, whole food, low insulin diet. Specifically, for PCOS, the insulin has got to be in check and doing well because high insulin (i.e., insulin resistance) is a key factor in throwing things off balance.[195,196]

With this understanding, you can see how all of the endocrine hormones work together and that the low insulin diet is not just for diabetics. It's necessary for any hormonal dysfunction so that the whole body can work well—it's the foundation that everyone needs to start with. You may need more testing and support based on the specifics of what is going on in your body, but keep in mind you can't out-supplement a bad diet.

I laid out the components of the low insulin diet and explained the whole thing to Kaylea and her husband, just as I did in this chapter. They were excited to get started, and she immediately shifted what they were eating. She

> You can't out-supplement a bad diet.

---

[195] https://www.ncbi.nlm.nih.gov/pmc/articles/PMC1334192/
[196] https://smile.amazon.com/PCOS-Plan-Prevent-Polycystic-Syndrome-ebook/dp/B084QBWCWQ/ref=sr_1_12?crid=1EJ6ZBP287YUA&keywords=pcos+diet&qid=1663882568&s=books&sprefix=pcos%2Cstripbooks%2C128&sr=1-12

soon started to feel more energized, even though she wasn't eating her usual fuel of carbohydrates. Within three months, she called to tell me that they were pregnant and ecstatic. I'm happy to say that they had a baby girl who is a good friend of my youngest daughter, as we were pregnant together during the process. There's no better resolution to a health concern than a baby, right?

Chapter 10
Talking About Toxins

Tessa came to see me after she found out that she had aggressive breast cancer, because she wanted to address things naturally. With cancer, there are always things that are driving it that absolutely must be addressed in order to get it into remission and ensure it won't return. Cancer doesn't just randomly happen—different parts of our terrains are imbalanced, and when too many areas are off, our body loses its designed ability to keep it in check.

So, we ran a series of tests to see what was out of whack for Tessa. One of the things that came back that surprised me was an extremely high level of benzene.

BECOMING TOXIN DETECTIVES

Benzene is an organic solvent that is a byproduct of industrial processes and combustion and comes from things such as vehicle exhaust, cigarette smoke, and outgassing of synthetic materials. It is mutagenic and carcinogenic and something that we wanted to look into further. While benzene is usually cleared out of the body within two days, we had to figure out where it was coming from, so that we could stop the inflow.

Tessa lives out in the middle of the country. There are no flight patterns above her, no highways, no exhaust fumes, and no huge number of synthetic materials. No one around her smokes, and nothing else pointed toward benzene. It can come through the ground water, but she already had good filters. We tested the water twice with and without the filter, and it was all fine. Our detective hats needed to come on because we were stumped.

About two months after we had started trying to figure this out, the tailpipe fell off her Jeep. When she took it in to the mechanic, he told her that the pipe that was connected to the tailpipe had several holes in it which were opening up into the cabin of her car.

Bingo! We had found the source, and it had been mitigated. There wasn't a strong enough odor for Tessa to be able to detect the benzene, but it had been a constant inflow of toxic, carcinogenic chemicals that she never would have known about if we hadn't run that test.

This was one piece of the puzzle for Tessa, and as we clicked her puzzle pieces together, she started to feel better.

One of the things that Tessa focuses on is heavy detoxification, including coffee enemas, infrared saunas, dry brushing, and rebounding. Getting her lymph flowing is imperative to helping her body rid itself of toxins and the excretion of the tumor breakdown.

Let me explain further. As blood circulates through your body, everything, except the red blood cells, exits the blood highway via the capillaries' off ramps. In the intercellular space, this plasma delivers the nutrients and picks up toxins, such as benzene, to be eliminated. It gets back on the blood highway by way of the lymph vessels. There are many lymph nodes on this path, which are like checkpoints for the truckers on our highways. There's lots of white blood cells, which are like the cops, that will look for and address any bad actors or toxins that are lurking about to ensure that they don't hurt your body. The lymph highway merges back into the blood highway around your heart, and from there, the toxins get filtered out by your liver or kidneys for excretion.[197]

Given this understanding, I was very glad that Tessa had not had surgery to remove those precious lymph nodes, or she wouldn't have been able to put the toxins we had found in containment. It would also have hindered her body in the detoxification that needed to happen.[198]

OTHER FORMS OF TOXINS

Suzanne came to me because she was having chronic explosive diarrhea. We started with the obvious gut work, but things really hadn't shifted as much as we were both hoping they would. She had also developed some new symptoms—she began having trouble walking. Suzanne was shuffling like an old man and could not walk anything but short distances.

But what concerned me the most was her brain fog. She couldn't remember conversations that she had just had, but what probably bothered her more was that she had stalled out on her weight loss, which had been going so well.

We decided to do some deeper testing. Unfortunately, my guess to look at a mold panel was right on, and we found that she had five times the acceptable range of verrucarin

---

[197] https://www.macmillan.org.uk/cancer-information-and-support/worried-about-cancer/the-lymphatic-system
[198] https://www.cancer.org/treatment/understanding-your-diagnosis/lymph-nodes-and-cancer.html

and elevated levels of sterigmatocystin, fumonisins, citrinin, and gliotoxin.

Once you have inhaled mold spores, they continue to poop toxins out and into you indefinitely (which is what gives you symptoms), so we didn't know if she was currently being exposed or if this was from an event in the past.[199] However, because her symptoms had shifted so dramatically during our work, I suspected this was a new issue and encouraged her to get a good mold inspector out to assess her house. The first guy said that there was no problem, but he didn't really do any testing, just a visual. I encouraged her to get a second opinion, and the next guy found several places in her house that had quite a bit of mold, including immense amounts in her air conditioning ducts.

Suzanne lives in Phoenix, which is not an area you would think of as being mold-laden because it is so dry. However, any place with an air conditioning system or water pipes that are hidden behind drywall (the perfect substrate to grow mold) are going to be at risk. (I keep trying to pitch the idea that we should have glass pipes on the outside of our walls so that we can see when there's a leak at any time—a kind of healthy, art deco look. So far no one's buying it though.)

Suzanne needed to make sure that she stopped the mold from coming into her house and her lungs before bothering to try to get it out of her body. She and her husband moved out while the mold remediation specialist took care of all these problems in a very controlled way. Then, she started a very robust protocol to address the mold spores that were in her

---

[199] https://smile.amazon.com/Break-Mold-Tools-Conquer-Health/dp/1988645182/ref=sr_1_1?crid=X92F60YTU7SF&keywords=jill+christa&qid=1663883277&s=books&sprefix=jill+christa%2Cstripbooks%2C197&sr=1-1

body. It included things such as an antifungal diet, binders for specific mold strains, daily infrared saunas, mitochondrial support, Omega-3s, bile flow support, anti-inflammatories and antioxidants, glutathione (not everyone can handle this with mold), antifungals, biofilm disruptors, and nebulized hydrogen peroxide.

Although the protocol was big, Suzanne did amazing! Within six months, her gait had returned to normal, and her brain was functioning at full capacity. She had even started losing weight again and had gone down two dress sizes. She finally felt like herself.

Because pipes can always leak, I encouraged her to watch for another exposure. Now, that she knew what her symptoms for mold were, it was a little easier to see them. Mold can have wide-ranging effects from what Suzanne had to things like fatigue, aches and pains, sinus problems, focusing issues, diarrhea, headaches, and mood swings.[200] These symptoms can masquerade as other issues and are hard to pin down, which is why you have to test. This is one of the tests that I always have my cancer clients run because it is so incredibly common.

We are bombarded by so many possibilities of being exposed to toxins and molds that it's almost rare not to find somebody who has some of these issues. It just depends how well you eliminate toxins, according to your individual genetics, combined with what you're eating and how you're living (epigenetics). All of this determines how you can withstand the onslaught. We're all different in how this plays out, which

---

[200] https://smile.amazon.com/Surviving-Mold-Life-Dangerous-Buildings-ebook/dp/B004NSVIYM/ref=sr_1_1?crid=1YK2HQJOW0NM1&keywords=shoemaker&qid=1663883427&s=books&sprefix=shoemaker%2Cstripbooks%2C181&sr=1-1

is why people can live in the same house and eat the same foods, and one gets cancer and the other doesn't.

Suzanne had quite a bit of excess weight when we started our work. There's a huge connection to high levels of toxins and weight gain. Suzanne tried every diet known (many I had not even heard of) and had a hard time losing weight. If she did manage to get some of it off, she gained it right back within months of going off the diet.

She did start a low insulin diet because we wanted to get the weight off. But with this kind of history, I suspected that there were going to be some toxins involved.

Here's the dirty secret about toxins—our body doesn't like toxic materials swirling around. If it knows that it isn't going to be able to get them out as fast as they're coming in, it puts them in our body's hazardous waste storage facilities. That's another name for fat.

Fat is where the body hides toxins so that they can't do as much damage to the rest of you. When trying to lose weight, your body is not going to want to release the fat stores if it knows that it's going to also be releasing toxic chemicals and metals that might swirl around and land in your brain, which is also made of fat.[201] If there are toxins that need to be addressed, the truth is that our bodies are actually protecting us by holding onto the weight.

> If there are toxins that need to be addressed, the truth is that our bodies are actually protecting us by holding onto the weight.

If there are toxins in the body—mycotoxins, heavy metals, non-metal toxins, and so on—you must support

---

[201] https://www.ncbi.nlm.nih.gov/pmc/articles/PMC6101675/

the detox process while trying to lose weight. They've got to go hand in hand.

First off, you absolutely must poop every day if you're going to try to do any of this work. It is also helpful to make sure that you fully digest all the nutrients that your body needs for the liver to package the toxins up for delivery out of your body. Support elimination routes with things like infrared saunas, coffee enemas, castor oil packs, rebounding, and dry brushing to ensure the process is successful.[202,203,204]

Once again, I want to give a shout out for the underutilized coffee enema. Besides being super cheap and easy, it also multitasks, which I always appreciate. Not only does it do the obvious of getting any backed-up poop out, but it also stimulates you into a parasympathetic state (key for those stuck in sympathetic/fight or flight), stimulates the liver to significantly increase the amount of glutathione (the body's mega-antioxidant), and stimulates the production and release of bile which also escorts toxins out of the body.[205,206,207]

I am the "Sam I Am" of coffee enemas—try them, try them, you will see, you will like them, just like me! I'm throwing down the gauntlet here—if you've got it in you, check out the QR code to my website NutritionalPilates.com at the end of the Introduction, which has all the directions to the best-kept health secret.

---

[202] https://www.ncbi.nlm.nih.gov/pmc/articles/PMC5941775/
[203] https://journals.physiology.org/doi/abs/10.1152/jappl.1980.49.5.881
[204] https://pubmed.ncbi.nlm.nih.gov/21168117/
[205] https://wellnessmama.com/health/coffee-enemas/
[206] https://draxe.com/health/coffee-enema/
[207] Son, Heejung, Hyun Jin Song, Hyun-Ju Seo, Heeyoung Lee, Sun Mi Choi, and Sanghun Lee. "The safety and effectiveness of self-administered coffee enema: A systematic review of case reports." *Medicine 99*, no. 36 (2020).

Detox Nutrients For The Liver

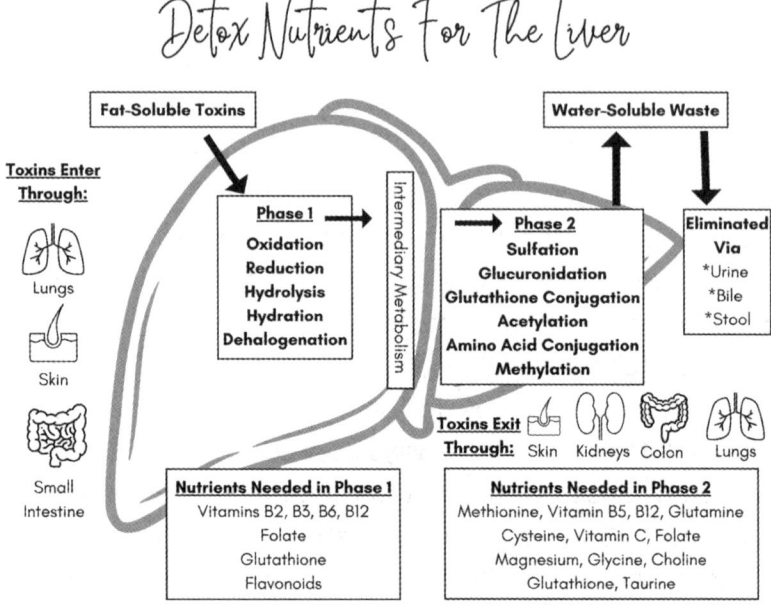

Figure 10-1: Detox nutrients for the liver

These are critical concepts that everyone needs to know because not only do we have a food system that is raising our insulin levels and causing us to gain weight, but we are also simultaneously being bombarded by toxins at an incredible level that has never been seen before in the history of humankind.

So many people dismiss needing to do detox work because they feel that, since we are designed to detox naturally a little every day, they are all set. While this is true, the level of toxins that we have daily exposure to is so high that we have to be proactive and work on this constantly to just tread water and not sink.[208,209]

---

[208] https://www.ewg.org/research/body-burden-pollution-newborns
[209] https://www.ncbi.nlm.nih.gov/pmc/articles/PMC6501744/

Chapter 11
Questions to Guide You on Your Journey

When I discovered I had cancer, I felt like I was free-falling. I knew that I didn't want what the oncologists were offering, but it was overwhelming and hard to figure out what I wanted to do. I didn't know who to turn to or who to trust, and it was scary. I felt very alone because most people thought I was crazy for going alternative in the first place. Besides my faith, the only thing that kept me going was looking at my kids' shining little faces and thinking about how they would feel if I didn't fight to be there on their wedding day.

I had to figure it out. It was all on me, and that was a huge weight, but there was enough fuel to keep me going in my search for answers on how to get my cancer in remission. Along the way, God graciously placed many beautiful people into my life who helped support and guide me through this process. I could not have gotten through that struggle without them!

Five Questions to Get You on Your Way

Now I want to pass along the hard questions that I struggled with in order to put my cancer into remission. There are five questions that I want you to ask yourself and honestly answer so that they can guide you to find your vibrance as well. Keep in mind that it is very easy to skip this section and avoid the application and implementation, but if you don't dig in and do the hard work, you won't get what you truly want.

What is your life going to look like if you make these huge changes?—I want you to use your imagination and picture what it looks like to shift your life in the ways we've discussed. What changes are you hoping for? How would these changes affect your daily life? How would they affect your relationships? What would that mean for you on a visceral, emotional level?

You might need some time to sit with this, to discuss this with someone you trust and feel safe with, or to journal about it in order to find your true motivation. I'll go first and share mine so you can get an idea of what I want you to explore.

For me, it isn't the short-term weight loss (although the postpartum mom in me would love that to hurry up!), it's the fact that I want to have my brain be as sharp as a tack and my body able to keep up with my grandkids when I'm eighty. I want to be the grandma that is out there running and playing with my grandkids (and maybe even my great-grandkids, if I'm truly blessed!)

When I had cancer, one of the things that broke my heart was that I might not get to teach my kids to ski. Now, I want to teach my grandkids to ski! I want to still be reading voraciously and learning new things constantly. This may be the most precious part of health to me—having a brain that can fire on all eight cylinders. I watched my father, who was an amazing visionary, gradually shut down over the last few decades until he couldn't even follow what he was watching on TV.

I have conquered cancer, and I have looked dementia straight in the eyes through my father—and I want no part of it. I am willing to skip the molten lava cake on my birthday if it means I get to know I'm having a birthday. I am okay with being the weird mom who is known to not want her receipts because they have xenoestrogens on them. I am honest about the fact that this will be an uphill battle based on what I know about how my body is wired.

One thing that I can guarantee is that it doesn't just "happen." Friends and clients make comments to the effect that it is easy for me—but it's not. I get tempted by favorite comfort foods, I want to fit in with everyone else, and I would love a nice treat when I have a bad day just as much as the next person. When I'm in those moments, I force myself to think about the bigger picture and what I'm working toward. That's my north star, and I want you to identify yours.

Who's your support?—I know that you understand how much of an impact the people in your life have on you. I want you to take inventory and evaluate each one of them. Determine who is going to be a positive, supportive influence in your life or a negative influence. Are they somebody that is going to lead you into temptation and away from your goals or belittle the choices you're making? Are there other ways that they would detract and pull you away from what you're creating?

It may take avoiding certain people for a time while you get stronger in your choices and make some progress. It may mean stepping outside of your comfort zone and asking a person in your life who is a positive influence for help or accountability.

This will look different for each one of you. Unfortunately, many people do not have the support systems that they need to make real change—this can make all the difference. If you don't have that support, please know that you can join our community and get your questions answered, be among other like-minded people, and get inspired with recipes, exercises, and tools to improve your health. We'll even let you join if you do have support because we can all use more love in our lives, right? This is where you can be reminded that you're not crazy, and what you're doing is important.

> "If you fail to plan, you're planning to fail."
>
> – BENJAMIN FRANKLIN

What changes do you want to make first?—Here's where the rubber meets the road. I want you to write down a list of what you learned that you want to apply. Name the change that you want to create by literally writing it down (or typing it). If you don't actually put your finger on it, it will just evaporate into nothingness as soon as you finish this book. You may want to set the book down right now and go do this. It's that important.

There are probably some areas of this book where you've felt some conviction and said: *Oh, that's me. I need to make that change.* Put those on your list, even if they're the hard ones that scare you, then put something at the top that is simple for you just to get the ball rolling and help you feel some success. There are a lot of psychological components to making lasting changes in your life, and what you choose to start with will make a big difference.

Quite frankly, there isn't a one-size-fits-all way to do this. Because you perfectionists are asking, "But what's the BEST change to start with?" here it is—it's the one that you're actually going to do. Start anywhere and make a change, then make another change, and another to get the ball rolling, one baby step at a time. Keep in mind that it is not about perfection but making more and more positive changes that will eventually shift how your body operates. Focus on upgrading your choices so it is a scale of good, better, best and not a black and white, or right and wrong, choice.

What is your plan to succeed in terms of food?—There are a lot of factors working against you in terms of eating well—you have to have your mental game on. Not only are almost all convenience foods and restaurants providing options that are working against you, but in most cases, you are going to be doing something different than your coworkers, friends, and family. Intentionality is what successful people have in common, so let's unpack it.

Please know that you're not special because you have kryptonite. We all do; we just need to know how to avoid it. No one is immune to the temptations of yummy food that is pretty much everywhere.

Now, living where I do—in the middle of nowhere—does have an advantage because there aren't billboards, fast-food restaurants, and access to junk food. However, when I go into town, it's there, and I always plan ahead of time what I will eat. Hot tip: planning to fast when going shopping never actually pans out so well.

If you see me on the street and ask nicely, I am happy to show you what's in my purse. What you would find is that I always carry at least one protein bar or fat bomb (but usually more, because little people are often inspired to hunger when they see Mom eating) and at least one special treat (usually chocolate if it's not in the heat of summer.)

Why? Because I know that when I am at a potluck or out somewhere where I can't get the outside-the-box food I need, that will be the time I'm likely to make bad choices that I'm going to regret later. I hate the whole dialogue in my head that goes, *Poor me, I have to do something weird, and I don't get to be like everybody else. I want to eat the yummy poison too!* Intentionality prevents me from attending the deprivation pity party.

I'm not going to lie to you—it is hard to be this intentional. You can't just fly by the seat of your pants, although I'm still praying that our food choices improve and good food becomes mainstream—a girl can dream, right? So, when our big family of nine travels, my trick is to hit up Costco (because they have pretty much the same things at all stores, have more organic and low carb options, and they are everywhere) and stay some place with a kitchen. Not only is this going to save us money, but it's also going to help us to be healthier so that we can actually enjoy our vacation without the meltdowns and mood imbalances that occur with junk food. If you're interested in seeing what we typically get for quick, throw-together, healthy meals with limited cooking resources (when camping or in hotel rooms) as well as our reusable shopping list, use the QR code at the end of the Introduction.

At home, creating a menu plan is key. Before you get anxious or close the book, I've got two different methods to this—there's something for everyone. The first method is traditional planning for the entire week (or month) with dishes precisely planned out and a shopping list created. There are plenty of sources for free online or you can pay a subscription to get new meal plans.

People love this because it is freeing to have the work of planning all done, but it isn't for everybody. Sometimes, this doesn't work if you are cooking from your garden, and it can be difficult if you have unusual food sensitivities.

I like to plan the day ahead. The night before, I will look at the produce that I have, see what needs to be eaten first and base the next day around that. I'll take meats out of the freezer that I'll need and soak or otherwise prep anything else that needs to be done ahead of time. I am still planning meals, but this allows me more creativity in the moment. I can see a recipe and try it the next day, and I still never end up wondering at 5 p.m. what we're going to eat. That's when things go sideways.

Note—with this method, you do have to keep your pantry and freezer stocked. This is a must for us living so far from the store, but it doesn't work for everyone. It's a personal preference as to how you plan, but you do need to plan.

You have to go against the norm if you want to be successful in health. Convenience foods are conveniently taking you toward chronic disease—if you want a different end result, you have to intentionally forge your own path. I know you can do this, or you wouldn't have made it this far through this book.

What is your plan to succeed in terms of movement?—If you were inspired to find your muscle imbalances and address them, let's make sure that you get a system in place to get the work done. When is it best for you to get some movement in? Many people like to work out first thing in the morning and that's fine if it works for you, but do not feel like you have to do what everyone else does. I often find that my best time to work out is after lunch, which goes against what most people prefer.

What tools do you have and what tools do you need? Do you want to work out at home or away from home? If you're working out at home, do you have items such as a foam roller, TheraBand, balls, mats, and hand weights? While you don't need these, they will give you more variety and may make the time more pleasurable if you're the type of person that gets bored easily. They may help you to address your muscle imbalances (i.e., things you suck at) with more variety by challenging them from different angles.

It is hard to work out at the gym if you don't have a membership. So, I'm stating the obvious here. Get everything set up and have a plan so that you can be intentional and strategic in addressing your muscle imbalances.

Do you need someone to help you assess your muscle imbalances or do you have a good idea of what you suck at? Working out by yourself is a fantastic way to go, but when you are looking at this new paradigm, you may want to have another pair of eyes to assess what your imbalances are and some direction on how to accomplish this.

Keep in mind that you are no longer limited to working with whoever is local—with technology, you can work out with people who are thousands of miles away. You need to be thoughtful about what you really want, because there are more choices than ever before.

These are questions that you want to take some time to consider. If you don't know all the dots from where you are now to where you want to go, how can you connect them with your daily choices? You can either use the resources I'm providing on our site, or you can apply the philosophy that I've presented to other disciplines, whatever you might be enjoying locally or online.

Conclusion

If you would like to find a professional to help you with either addressing your muscle imbalances or the low insulin diet, I want to give you some ideas of what to look for in a practitioner so that you can be as successful as possible. Unfortunately, in both of these disciplines there is a huge spectrum of skill. The key is to ask the right questions when you are looking for someone. Most importantly, you want someone you gel with—this is an intangible thing to quantify, but at its heart is trust and respect. Do you respect who they are and what they do? Do you trust that they can help you and that you'll benefit from working with them?

Beyond that, with Pilates, you want to look for a practitioner who is able to identify and work with muscle imbalances (this is not always included in basic training); that way, they can tailor the work to you. If you ask them about this and they have no idea what you're talking about, then they are not the practitioner for you.

You want someone who is able to clearly express what they want you to do or not do, and why. It is important to have someone who can work with the equipment that you have or is close to you so that you can work with the equipment that they have. (This could be on Zoom or in person, depending on what you prefer.) You want somebody who has experience to work with any conditions that you may have. I also recommend that you look for someone who has training experience with both contemporary and classical Pilates—this is going to give them an open mind and a breadth of understanding that's going to be far superior to either one on its own.

When looking for a functional nutritionist, you want someone who understands the body beyond just the government mis-guidelines. Ask them what types of diets they work with, and if they aren't familiar with a low insulin diet, you might want to look elsewhere. You don't want someone who is stuck on one diet and isn't comfortable personalizing it to each client.

It is also important for practitioners to have done these diets themselves because then they will know how to problem-solve, how to cook that way, and how to answer your questions.

Of course, you'll want a practitioner who has experience working with any medical conditions that you may have in a functional perspective. Look for a practitioner who has the ability to read, interpret, and order functional tests, including Great Plains ENVIROtox Complete, DUTCH testing, DiagnosTechs cycling hormone panels, Vibrant panels, GI map or GI360, Cyrex panels, Nutrition Genome, or 3x4 Genetics testing.

It's important to ask a practitioner what their personal health journey has been, when and how they overcame their health struggles, and what kinds of things they currently do for their health.

You'll also want to know how much ongoing continuing education they partake in on a regular basis. There are so many cutting-edge discoveries and theories coming out daily that practitioners really need to stay on top of to be as helpful as possible to their clients. Their answers will show you how thoroughly they are going to be able to help you, what kind of resources they have, and how much empathy they will have for what you are going through.

There is no magic bullet. Reread that last sentence a few times. Most people who have a condition, an issue, or a pain want to go to a practitioner who gives them a single supplement or prescription to make it go away, but it just doesn't work that way. I'm sorry to say this because I, too, wish it did.

> There is no magic bullet.

When you're focused on looking for the magic bullet, you miss the bigger picture. It took you a long time to get into this mess by making many misdirected lifestyle and diet choices, and it's going to take a little while to unravel this knotted-up ball of yarn that you have.

If you choose to work with a practitioner, you want somebody who is going to customize things to you, not someone who's just going to throw you a one-size-fits-all solution, no matter what their marketing promises. And if you chase the magic bullet, keep in mind that "Band-Aid" medications or supplements usually do not solve the problem, even if they do fix one symptom. You've got to get to the root issue of why the body is manifesting those indicators of imbalance. This must start with addressing symptoms and what they're pointing to, not just covering them up.

When I had cancer, I did not even realize that I had symptoms, much less that they would manifest into something crazy! I mean, come on—I was thirty-eight and felt fine!

When I met the practitioner who helped me address my cancer, I was hesitant. I wanted to give her a chance; I needed to give her a chance, but I felt guarded. It wasn't until we worked together for a while that I knew that she had my best interests at heart, she really cared about me, and she had the tools and background to help guide me through the process.

If I had known then what I'm sharing with you now, I would have known what questions to ask so that I could trust her more from the beginning. During the functional lab tests, it became apparent that she knew what she was talking about and that these were the right tools to show me how I had gotten into this hot mess. That's when I started to feel empowered—when I understood the *why* behind what was going on, I knew that there was a path to correct it and furthermore, to prevent it from recurring.

Going through that process not only made me feel empowered, but it also excited me to see firsthand how our bodies are able to heal themselves, and I wanted to learn more! As soon as I was in the clear, I signed up for an entry level nutrition training program, and from there, went into functional lab training and later, specialized cancer training. I wanted to do the work that my practitioner had done with me. I wanted to help other people and share the vision that our bodies are designed to heal.

Remember Tessa, who I'm working with on her breast cancer? Well, she is actually a close friend of mine who supported me when I was sick and going the alternative medicine route. I now have the privilege of supporting her as her practitioner as she walks her own cancer journey.

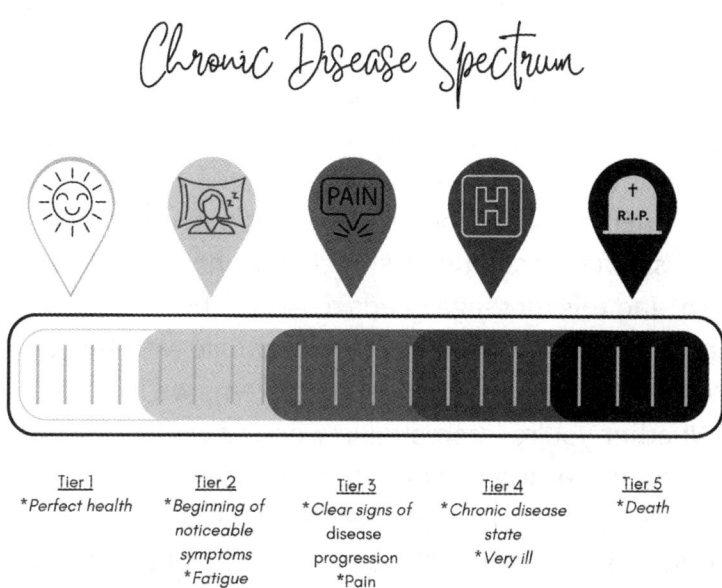

Figure 4-1: Chronic disease spectrum from Chapter 4

Do you know where you are on the chronic disease spectrum? Do you have some niggling symptoms that are pointing toward your future or are you already there and you want to back things up and get yourself into remission? Identifying where you are is going to give you a lot of great insight as to how much work you're going to need to do and how urgent it is that you do it.

Do you remember when I asked you at the beginning what type of person you were? If you're the frugal DIY person, then you're probably already applying parts of this book, researching other ideas that I've discussed, and you might already have what you need. If you're the person who needs some help, please know that there are lots of practitioners out there who can do this work. My team at Nutritional Pilates loves the opportunity to guide others through their journey to vibrant health. And if you want to work with me personally, check out the intimate Nutritional Pilates Retreat that I run biannually.

If you're the person who wants to learn to help yourself while you create a new flexible career at the same time, I would like to extend a personal invitation to you to join our practitioner training program. The world needs more altruistic, passionate practitioners! Each of us has power over our health, and this message needs to get further out there than I can do alone. We need to arm the public with this understanding if we want to change the systems we live in.

Whether you're interested in working with a practitioner or becoming a practitioner, go ahead and check out the resources on our site with the QR code at the end of the Introduction (also shown below) or check out our website at NutritionalPilates.com.

https://nutritionalpilates.com/step/book-resources-optin/

I challenge you to take action because the world needs more people who understand that the body was designed for health. I want to thank you so much for taking the time to read this book, and my prayers are with you on your journey to discover a new level of health!

About the Author

Katrina is an educator, an author, and an international presenter. She is board certified in holistic nutrition and is a second-generation Pilates Master Teacher. Her passion is teaching, which she has been doing for over twenty years—Pilates teacher training as well as functional lab training for practitioners. Katrina and her team work with clients all over the world, helping people reclaim their health and reverse chronic disease.

But her favorite credentials are her seven kids! Katrina and her family live in rural Idaho on 15 acres where they raise cows and chickens along with organic produce. She is passionate about practicing what she preaches and is continually working to improve her health and the health of her family.

You can learn more about Katrina at www.Nutritional-Pilates.com/about or by following her on Instagram @katrinafoe or on Facebook at www.facebook.com/nutritional.pilates